Cataracts

BY JULIUS SHULMAN, M.D.

Cataracts
No More Glasses

Cataracts

REVISED EDITION

Julius Shulman, M.D.

Illustrations by Neil Hardy

ST. MARTIN'S GRIFFIN
NEW YORK

Design by Helene Berinsky

All illustrations © 1993 Neil O. Hardy

Library of Congress Cataloging-in-Publication Data

Shulman, Julius
    Cataracts / Julius Shulman. — Rev. ed.
      p.   cm.
    Includes index.
    ISBN 0-312-13039-2
    1. Cataract—Popular works. I. Title.
RE451.S54   1995
617.7'42—dc20   95-44032
                                   CIP

First St. Martin's Griffin Edition: July 1995

10 9 8 7 6 5 4 3 2

To my wife, Shelli,
children, Ilana, Lauren, Michael;
and to my father and to my mother, who,
perhaps, can somehow read this

Acknowledgments

It is with immense gratitude and appreciation that I thank the late Barbara Bannon, whose guidance and support were a catalyst for this book. My friend Jethro Lieberman, a.k.a. W. M., abetted this undertaking and taught me some writing along the way. Thanks also to Florence Janover of Sensible Solutions who helped get this second edition into print. And a special thanks to Dr. Robert Coles, who was a role model for me and all physicians who strove to be good doctors and good to their patients.

Contents

Preface

If you are reading this book, chances are that you have or someone close to you has a cataract. Perhaps you are contemplating cataract surgery or have had an operation already. Since almost 1½ million cataract operations are performed each year in the United States alone, you are in good company. This book will help you understand the nature of cataracts and cataract surgery—whether to have an operation and, if so, what type. The technological revolution in eye surgery has made it difficult for the layperson to understand the different types of cataract surgery and arrive at an intelligent and correct decision. Cataract surgery, more than any other type of surgery, requires important decisions from the patient, since the decision to undergo surgery depends on how poorly you see and how your eyesight limits your daily activities. If you have already had surgery, this book should answer many of your questions that may have been left unresolved. It will also aid you in getting through those first few postoperative weeks, when your sight may change constantly, your eye may be a source of anxiety and apprehension, and things may actually seem worse before they get better. Rest assured, though. The success rate for cataract surgery is over 95 percent, so the chances are excellent that you will fully regain your sight.

1

What Is a Cataract?

**"Your vision is blurred because
you have cataracts."**

The diagnosis of cataract is made by ophthalmologists throughout the world hundreds of times every day. Cataracts are one of the most common afflictions known. In its early stages a cataract is not a disease at all, but a normal part of aging. It is one of the world's leading causes of blindness and although it is more common among older people, it can even be present at birth. If we live long enough, almost all of us will develop cataracts.

A cataract is a loss of transparency, or clouding, of the normally clear lens of the eye. In order to see sharply and clearly, light must pass into our eye through a crystal-clear lens, just as a sharply focused picture depends on light passing through a clear camera lens. As we age chemical changes occur in the human lens that render it less transparent. The loss of transparency may be so mild as to hardly affect vision, or be so severe that no shapes or movements are seen, only light and dark. When the lens gets cloudy enough to obstruct vision to any significant degree, it is called a cataract.

The origin of the word cataract is fascinating though somewhat obscure, stemming from misconceptions during Greek and Roman times that cataracts were evil liquids that flowed into the eye. A papyrus dating to 1500 B.C. describes what was probably a cataract under the phrase "the mounting of water in the eye." The Greeks used the words *hypochyma* and *hypochysis*, meaning "water underneath," while the Romans used the Latin term *suffusis* to describe a cataract as a suffusion, or overspreading. During the Middle Ages the Arabs translated the term for cataract into an Arabic word meaning "black water." Later that Arabic word was translated back into Latin as the word *cataracta*—a waterfall. The Latin *cataracta* became the English cataract.

Although cataracts were recognized more than 3,000 years ago, it took centuries for doctors and scientists to begin to understand the nature and causes of this malady. Learned scholars such as Leonardo da Vinci (1452–1519) and Andreas Vesalius (1514–1564) staunchly maintained that a cataract was an evil humor or phlegm that covered and clouded the front of the lens, rather than a disease of the lens itself.

Credit goes to Warner Rolfink (1599–1673), an anatomy professor in Jena, Germany, for first publishing the true nature of a cataract. Rolfink learned of the French surgeon François Quarre, who believed that a cataract was merely a clouded lens. By the gruesome task of dissecting the eyes of executed criminals (of which there were plenty), Rolfink confirmed his theory.

In order to understand what's going on inside the eye and how the lens turns cloudy, you have to learn more about the human lens. The next chapter describes the workings of the whole eye, but for now let's get a good foundation for understanding a cataract—starting with the lens.

The *lens* is a transparent organ about the size of a pea that sits just behind the *iris*, the colored part of your eye. (See Fig. 1.) There are three parts to the lens: the *capsule*, the *nucleus*, and the *cortex*. The capsule is a thin membrane that completely surrounds the lens, much like the skin of a peach. When we are young, the center of the lens, the nucleus, is soft, almost the consistency of custard. As we get older, into our fifties and sixties, the nucleus gets sclerotic, or hard, somewhat resembling the pit of a peach. The rest of the lens, the cortex, is made up of long, arching fibers, running from top to bottom, similar to the fruit of a peach (Fig. 1). As we age, the older fibers are pushed to the center of the lens and compacted, while the newer, looser fibers are near the outside. To switch analogies, the growth of the lens resembles that of a tree—both continue to grow throughout life with the older part in the center and the newer parts on the outside.

The function of the lens is to refract, or bend, light rays to focus them to a clear image on the back of the eye. The lens, being somewhat elastic, will change shape to focus light properly, automatically getting fatter for close objects, such as the type on this page, and thinner for distant objects, such as a street sign. Starting as early as age twenty, the lens slowly loses its elasticity, until at around age forty or forty-five it cannot change shape enough to

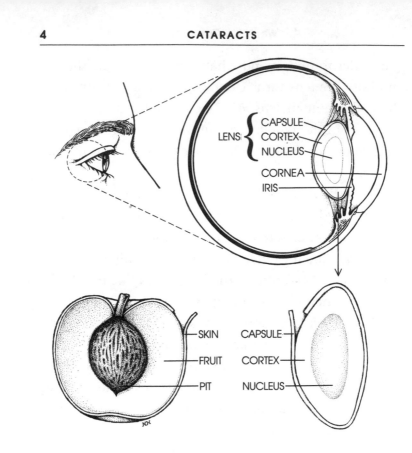

Figure 1   The human lens is compared to a peach.

bring close objects into focus. Reading glasses, that inevitable admission of "middle age," will then be necessary to
aid in focusing. The shape of the lens is automatically
controlled by the *ciliary muscle*, a thin band of muscle that
lines the wall of the eye.

The ciliary muscle surrounds the lens like a headband
and is connected to it by *zonules*, thin jellylike strands that

suspend the lens in place like strings suspending a puppet. Although each zonule is weak by itself, the suspensory framework formed by thousands of them is amazingly strong. Severe or repeated head trauma, such as that sustained by boxers, or by people in automobile accidents, is sometimes enough to disrupt the zonules and dislodge the lens from its normal position. The result of such trauma is often a cataract.

The lens has the highest protein content of any organ in the body, 33 percent compared to 18 percent for muscle. You can cut a T-bone steak as thin as you possibly can and yet you will not be able to see through it, but the lens is easily transparent although it has almost twice the protein content of steak. The reason for this transparency is the unique physical and chemical orderly arrangement of the protein fibers in the lens, as opposed to the more variable, disorderly arrangement of fibers in steak or any nontransparent part of our body. If even a very small part of the lens gets cloudy enough to block rays of light— whether it is the central nucleus, the outer cortex, or the thin surrounding capsule—that part is called an *opacity*. If enough opacities form in the lens to affect vision, or if a general loss of transparency occurs, the end result is a cataractous lens—a cataract. A cataract is not a skin or a film over the eye, nor is it a growth or infection. It is merely a loss of transparency of the normally clear lens. The more cloudy the lens and the more the center of the lens is involved, the worse the vision.

To better understand cataracts, we must review how the eye works.

2

How the Eye Sees

The Parts of the Eye

A simple explanation of how the eye sees is that the eye does not do the seeing, the brain does. In fact, the eye is really an extension of the brain, and gathers information for processing in much the same way as a TV antenna gathers a signal for processing by the picture tube of a television. We need to examine each part of the eye in order to get a better understanding of the vision process.

If you look at your eye in a mirror, the most obvious feature is its color. This comes from a pigmented structure called the *iris*. (See Fig. 2.) We are all born with lightly colored eyes. If the iris becomes very pigmented, we wind up with brown eyes. The less the pigment, the bluer your eyes will be. If you look a little more closely, you will see a black hole in the middle of the iris. This is the pupil, the opening through which light travels into your eye. The pupil controls the amount of light that enters the eye, becoming smaller in bright light and larger in dim light.

If you take a flashlight and shine it into your eye while looking at the pupil in a mirror, you will see the constant adjustment in pupil size as light hits your eye. What you probably cannot see is a sparkling-clear dome-shaped membrane that vaults over the front of the eye like a

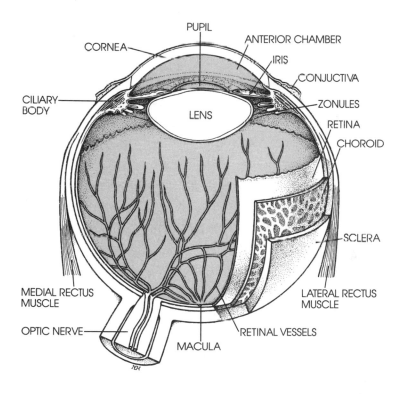

Figure 2 The parts of the eye.

skylight on a roof. This is the *cornea*, and clear vision is as much dependent on a clear cornea as on a clear lens. When a foreign body hits your eye it seems to invariably land on the cornea, whose rich supply of pain fibers makes you feel as if sandpaper were trapped under your eyelids. The *sclera*, the white of the eye, surrounds the cornea and extends completely around the eye, giving it strength and substance.

A thin membrane, the *conjunctiva*, covers the white of the eye and lines the inside of the lids. The conjunctiva has tiny blood vessels that, with mild infection, allergy, or pollution, can become enlarged, causing the eye to look bloodshot. Conjunctivitis, or pinkeye, results when this layer becomes infected.

Working together, the cornea, the pupil, and the lens focus light onto the back of the eye, the *retina*. This is a thin, diaphanous membrane that lines the inside of the back of the eye. The retina, which can be compared to the film in a camera, "takes" the picture, and the brain "develops" it. The retina sends the picture to the brain by way of a thick nerve in the back of the eye, the *optic nerve*. As illustrated in Figure 2, the eye has an inner layer, the retina, as well as an outer layer, the *sclera*. The middle layer, the *choroid*, is rich in blood vessels and darkly pigmented, resembling the skin of a grape. In fact, another name for the choroid is the uvea, which means "grape" in Latin. This uvea forms the iris in the front of the eye and the choroid in the back of the eye. Most of the blood circulation that nourishes the eye travels in the choroid.

Two other parts deserve mention, since they make up

the fluid portion of the eye. The space between the iris and cornea, called the *anterior chamber*, is filled with *aqueous*, a solution resembling spinal fluid. New aqueous fluid is constantly being formed to replace aqueous that filters out of the eye. A blockage of this fluid results in elevated pressure in the eye—glaucoma. Most of the inside cavity of the eye is filled with the *vitreous*, a jellylike material that gives the eye substance and volume. "Floaters," those annoying black spots we commonly see, are protein particles that float in the vitreous.

How We See

Let's see what happens, from front to back, when a ray of light enters your eye. How is a painting transformed from a mixture of oils, pigments, and canvas to a picture of color, texture, depth, and warmth in your brain? Each part of the eye plays a role.

Light bouncing off a painting or a tree or a book will first hit your cornea, the clear dome-shaped front part of your eye. The image will now be about 60 percent focused as the cornea bends (refracts) the rays of light. Light then passes through the pupil and enters the lens, which bends the rays of light another 40 percent. In the ideal situation this should result in an image focused to a sharp point on the retina. The light acts like an electric shock through the ten layers of cells in the retina and stimulates them to send their message to the brain. Most of the light is focused on an area of the retina called the *macula*, where vision is the sharpest and clearest. It is this "central vision," supplied by retinal cells called cones, that allows us to read, watch a movie, or drive a car. The rest of the retina, populated by cells called rods, gives peripheral, or side, vision, also important in driving a car and generally getting around. Without peripheral vision we would be left with only "tunnel vision" and would constantly collide with objects in our path. The cones, which are mostly active in vision during daylight, also supply us with color vision. There are cones for red, yellow, and blue; how we appreciate the hundreds of colors in our environment via cells for only the three primary colors is truly amazing and still not completely understood.

If the light rays were always focused to a sharp point on the retina, we would never need glasses. We need glasses, or have a refractive error, when this point of focus falls in front of the retina, as in myopia (nearsightedness), or behind the retina, as in hyperopia (farsightedness). In spite of its complexity, the retina merely sends to the brain whatever image it receives, clear or blurred. Glasses correct the refractive error and clear up the blurred image by focusing the rays of light onto the retina. Astigmatism, from the Greek *a*, meaning "without," and *stigma*, meaning "point," results when the image is not focused to a point at all, usually because of an irregularly shaped cornea. Glasses for astigmatism first have to bend the light rays to a point, whether in front of or in back of the retina, and then bring this point to a sharp focus on the retina itself.

Vision is measured using the familiar Snellen chart,

which has lines of increasingly smaller numbers. Developed in 1864 by the Dutch ophthalmologist, Herman Snellen, each line of the chart corresponds to a different level of vision, such as 200, 100, 70, 40, and 20, which is somewhat arbitrarily designated as "normal." The vision of each eye is expressed as a fraction: The top number represents the testing distance from the chart, commonly 20 feet, and the bottom number represents the smallest line the patient can see. If while standing 20 feet from the chart, your right eye can see only the larger letters such as the "85" of the 200 line, the vision in your right eye would be designated 20/200. (See Fig. 3.) (Compared to the weak 20/200 eye, a normal, 20/20 eye would be able to see the 200 line on the eye chart from as far away as 200 feet.) If one eye sees 20/20 and the other eye, the one

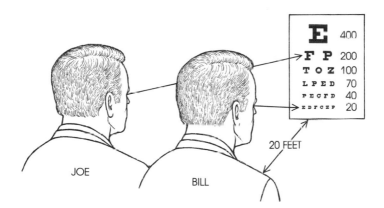

Figure 3　From 20 feet away, Bill can see the small letters on the 20 line, while Joe can see only the large letters of the 200 line. Bill has 20/20 vision; Joe has 20/200 vision. (By definition, with 20/20 vision, Bill can see the 20 line from 20 feet as well as the 200 line from 200 feet.)

with a cataract, sees 20/100, the total vision of the person with both eyes open would still be 20/20. This is a very important point for patients with a cataract in one eye and a normal, clear lens in the other eye. A cataract does not have to be removed just because it's there. We'll learn more about that in Chapter 7.

Now that we know what a cataract is and how the normal eye sees, let's get to what brings you to the eye doctor in the first place—the symptoms of a cataract.

3

Symptoms of a Cataract

"I'm not sure I'm seeing as I used to. I keep thinking my glasses are dirty and things just don't seem right."

"When I look at TV I get a double image. I see two televisions instead of one!"

"I'm getting better in my old age. I don't need my reading glasses anymore!"

"What's the matter with my doctor? He's given me three pairs of glasses in the last six months and I'm still not seeing right!"

"Bright lights make me so blurred I can't even cross the street on a sunny day. I don't see how it's possible, but I see better on a cloudy day."

"Colors don't seem as bright as they used to—everything seems kind of yellow, like there's a film over my eye."

All these complaints are commonly voiced by patients

with symptoms of a cataract. Since most symptoms start slowly and gradually, many patients accept the changes in vision as a normal accompaniment of aging, and don't feel compelled to see their ophthalmologist until their vision is quite blurred. Let's examine cataract symptoms one by one.

The first complaint is the most common symptom of a cataract: You are not seeing as well as you used to. The degree to which you notice this symptom varies, depending on how sensitive you are to a change in vision. This may be so subtle and gradual (over many months and years) as to confuse patient and doctor alike. The change in vision often starts with a vague, nagging feeling, a slight inkling, that something is wrong with your sight. Initially there may be no supporting objective findings— you may still be measured as 20/20—but that clock across the street may not seem as clear as it did six months ago. You keep thinking your glasses are dirty, your eyes are tired. If you are particularly sensitive to slight vision changes, or your work involves fine detail, such as that done by an engineer or a designer, a typical visit to your ophthalmologist may contain the following:

PATIENT: Doctor, something is wrong. I'm not seeing right.

DOCTOR: Well, I checked your vision and it's still 20/20, or just about. And you don't need any change in glasses; that won't help. I do detect some very early changes in the lens of your eyes, but you are seventy-three years old and this is probably normal aging rather than true cataracts. The rest of your eye examination is perfectly normal, so let me check you again in about six months. Please call me if anything develops before that.

Another patient may not notice changes in vision until a cataract is fairly advanced, or may have subconsciously denied health symptoms as many of us do because of fear or anxiety. In that case the visit may take place much later and be entirely different:

PATIENT: Doctor, something is wrong. I'm not seeing right.

DOCTOR: I'm surprised you've gone this long. You definitely have cataracts and will soon need cataract surgery.

Each patient reacted differently to the symptoms; one was sensitive to a slight change in vision and the other waited until the diminished vision was more noticeable.

Seeing double, another cataract symptom, may be caused by an eye-muscle problem, such as crossed eyes or a wandering eye, or by a cataract that is not uniformly dense or opaque. One part of the lens may have more opacities than another, causing rays of light, such as from a TV screen, to split into two or even three different parts. This is especially true of a small cataract in the nucleus, the central hard part of the lens. Here is an easy test to determine if double vision is from a cataract: Cover the good eye and see if the double vision disappears. If it does, the cataract is not causing double vision and most likely the eye muscles are at fault, causing your eyes to be misaligned. Although eye muscle trouble, such as crossed eyes, is more common in children and usually means nothing more serious than muscle imbalance, eye muscle trouble in adults often stems from neurologic problems. Double vision in the bad eye, on the other hand—which would persist with the good eye covered—may well be caused by a cataract, and a visit to the ophthalmologist will help diagnose your problem.

The third cataract symptom, the newly acquired ability to read without glasses, is another common symptom of cataracts, and the understandable enthusiasm for this "second sight" belies a developing cataract. The explanation lies in the part of the lens first affected by the cataractous process. As we learned in Chapter 2, the lens is divided into three parts—an outer capsule, an inner central nucleus, and the fibers in between, the cortex. If the cataract starts in the central nuclear area, the nucleus will become hard or sclerotic, the same way cholesterol deposits in arteries cause hardening of the arteries, or arteriosclerosis. When the nucleus becomes hard, the lens gets fatter and optically stronger, so that light will be focused in front of the retina. The net effect on the eye is that it becomes nearsighted, causing near objects to be in focus even without reading glasses or bifocals. Becoming nearsighted or less farsighted, and perhaps not needing glasses to read at all, may be the earliest and the only clue to the presence of a developing cataract. In fact, at this stage the lens in your eye may not look cataractous at all but may appear completely normal. Patients who are already severely nearsighted may develop markedly reduced vision from a very small cataract, one that would not bother a patient who was not severely nearsighted.

Nearsightedness from a developing cataract also explains the necessity for frequent changes of eyeglasses. As the cataract increases your nearsightedness, the eyeglass prescription must keep pace with the changes in your eye. Although this may be a nuisance, you should realize how fortunate you are in being able to maintain your usual level of vision by merely changing your glasses. As the cataract matures, however, glasses will no longer maintain your sight and surgery will eventually be necessary.

Poor vision in bright light and improved vision in dim light may seem paradoxical at first. If a cataract cuts down on the light entering the eye, shouldn't more light help? The answer depends on the type of cataract and which part of the lens is affected. When most of the clouding is centered on the back or posterior surface of the lens, the cataract will have its greatest impact when the pupil, or opening into the eye, is small. When, as would happen on a sunny day, the small pupil directly corresponds in size and shape to the clouded center of the lens, like something blocking the bull's-eye of a target, vision will be quite blurred. The brighter the light, the smaller the pupil, and the worse the vision. This type of cataract, technically called a posterior subcapsular (PSC) cataract, is more common in patients with diabetes and in patients on long-term use of cortisone, such as those with severe arthritis or asthma. The bull's-eye effect may be quite incapacitating to a patient with even a relatively small PSC cataract, since the level of vision, or visual acuity, may be markedly reduced on anything other than a cloudy day. Drops to keep the pupil dilated may improve vision temporarily until cataract surgery is performed. The problem may not even be readily apparent in the ophthalmologist's office, because most of the time the room is fairly dark when vision is tested. Should your ophthalmologist detect a PSC cataract, or any cataract producing excessive glare, your vision should be retested with the room lights on; this will give a more realistic assessment of your diminished eyesight.

Your ophthalmologist may take this one step further by using a Brightness Acuity Test (BAT) or similar glare device. During this test you read the eye chart while increasingly strong light shines into your eye, simulating bright sunshine. A dramatic decrease in vision with bright light may indicate that cataract surgery is needed in spite of relatively good vision on the eye chart.

Ophthalmologists assess not only visual acuity but your visual function, or how you function with your level of vision. Acceptable vision on the eye chart and unacceptable vision in daily life, which can include difficulty with reading or driving or in other situations involving glare, may exist simultaneously; recommending cataract surgery to such a patient is often more an art than a science. In the past, eye doctors would wait until your vision dropped to levels as low as 20/70 or even 20/100 before advising cataract surgery, but with modern, safer surgery and more rapid recovery (as we shall see in Chapter 9), patients can have cataract surgery earlier. Now, doctors rely less and less on visual acuity and more on visual function, weighing this against the traditional "risk-benefit ratio" in recommending surgery.

The last symptom of a cataract, a change in color vision, is a subtle alteration in the quality of your vision that may be overshadowed by more noticeable alterations in its clarity. As the cataract progresses, the nucleus becomes more and more yellow. In becoming yellower, the cataract absorbs wavelengths of first violet and then blue light, effectively reducing those colors and making the environment appear yellowish. The opposite effect often occurs immediately after cataract surgery, when a flood of blue and violet light enters the eye and everything looks blue.

The underlying theme that runs through all the symptoms of a cataract is that your eyesight is getting worse. The change is usually quite gradual and painless and occurs over months and years. Lights may cause glare, colors may look yellow, you may sense a film over your eyes, but the dominant problem is that you just can't see as well as you used to. If a cataract develops in only one eye and that is your nondominant eye, you may not even know it is there until the vision in that eye is surprisingly poor.

Most people not only have a dominant hand that makes them a "rightie" or a "leftie," but also a dominant eye that gives them more comfortable vision despite equal vision with their nondominant eye. To find your dominant eye, bring together the tip of your thumb and forefinger into an "O," about six inches from your face. It is important to keep both eyes open. Focus on an object across the room so that it is in the middle of the "O." Closing

one eye and then the other will tell you which eye is
dominant. If you close your left eye and the object is still
in the center of the "O," then your right eye was the
"sighting" eye and is the dominant one and vice versa. If
a choice were possible, it would be better to have a cataract
in your nondominant eye, because good vision in your
dominant eye will feel more comfortable and natural. An
ophthalmologist I know developed a cataract in his dominant, right eye, but deferred surgery for a while because
his left eye was still 20/20. Only after cataract surgery
restored 20/20 vision in his dominant eye did he really
feel he could see again.

What causes cataracts to develop? In the next chapter
we'll discuss some of the reasons cataracts are so common.

4

What Causes Cataracts?

Age is the major predisposing cause of cataracts. Some loss of transparency of the lens will happen to all of us if we live long enough. The resulting change in the lens, if significant, is called a *senile cataract*. The word senile comes from the Latin word for "old" and has nothing to do with mental faculties or behavior. Cataracts are part of the price we pay for our increasing longevity. In much the same way, aging will cause our hair to gray, our hearing to diminish, and our joints to develop arthritis.

Of the 2 million people in the United States with visually disabling cataracts, well over 90 percent have senile cataracts. The majority of people in their seventies and eighties show some mild cataractous changes. Since these changes generally do not significantly affect vision, they would not be termed true cataracts, but just normal changes in the lens due to age. The lens may be a little yellow or cloudy, and vision may be somewhat reduced by one or two lines on the eye chart. This change in vision need not and probably will not significantly interfere with reading, driving, watching television, and taking part in most other daily activities.

A study done in 1968 in the United States showed that more than 80 percent of people over age sixty-five had some lens clouding attributable to age. Another study, the Health and Nutrition Examination Survey conducted by the Department of Health, Education and Welfare and reported in the *Archives of Ophthalmology* in April 1982, specifically looked for cataracts and vision loss in the older population. Of the thousands of people studied between sixty-five and seventy-five years of age, better than 30 percent had cataracts. In other words, of every ten people sixty-five years or older, about eight will show some aging change in the lens of each eye, and at least three will have diminished vision due to cataracts. The important finding to emerge from these and other studies is that if you or someone you know is sixty-five years or older, there is an 80 percent chance of the very beginning of a cataract and a 30 percent chance of some vision loss from a cataract. Cataracts are a very common condition and, until now, a normal and inevitable part of the aging process. In later chapters, we discuss the possibility of actually preventing cataract formation. Your ophthalmologist will be able to examine your eyes and tell you if cataracts are developing.

But if cataracts are a normal part of the aging process, why is there so much variation among individuals? Why can an eighty-year-old have only mild vision problems, while his sixty-nine-year-old brother has already had surgery for advanced cataracts? Why are some babies born with cataracts? Why will a cataract take ten years to grow in one eye and only one year to grow in the other eye of the same person? The answer, at present, is that we just don't know. Many factors have been implicated in causing senile cataracts, from lack of vitamins to prolonged exposure to ultraviolet light, but until recently no conclusive evidence of any kind has been found. Intensive investigation is being conducted throughout this country, not only in the laboratory but in doctors' offices and hospital clinics.

Jules Stein, M.D., the famous musical entrepreneur who founded the Music Corporation of America, established Research to Prevent Blindness, a New York–based philanthropy devoted to research in eye disease and ending blindness, no matter what the cause. A great deal of cataract eye research is supported by this organization, as well as by the National Institutes of Health and other private and governmental agencies. The impetus for this research is partly financial. It is estimated that almost $5 billion will be spent in 1995 in treating cataract patients in the United States alone.

A Probable Cause

What is finally emerging as one probable cause of cataracts is damage to the lens by oxidation, the same process that causes iron to rust and the pages of an old book to yellow. Oxidation, a normal part of our metabolism occurring throughout the body, has been implicated in causing not only cataracts, but many disorders, including cancer and heart disease. Oxidation releases chemicals called free radicals that, in the heart, can turn cholesterol rancid and clog your arteries. In the eye, the sources of oxidation or oxidative stress, the scientific term, include ultraviolet radiation (UV light), x-radiation (X ray), and even the cosmic radiation to which our astronauts are exposed. Because the front of the eye is so transparent, the lens is constantly bathed in light, including ultraviolet light, and over many years the delicate protein arrangement in the lens gets damaged. Transparency, an all-important property of the lens, suffers and vision becomes blurred. Ultraviolet light, the part of sunlight responsible for a suntan, can be as harmful to the eye as it is to the skin. Soviet astronauts, exposed to high levels of cosmic radiation 300 miles above the earth, are now reported to be showing signs of cataracts. American astronauts are also at risk, although they have orbited only 150 to 200 miles above the earth. If research implicating UV light as a cause of cataracts proves to be true, the predicted 10 percent depletion of the earth's ozone layer over the next ten years will, according to a 1991 United Nations panel of scientists, result in almost 2 million new cataract cases worldwide. Our increased exposure to ultraviolet light, normally filtered by ozone in the stratosphere, will result not only in more cataracts, but in more skin cancer and weakened immunity.

Although little doubt now exists that cataract formation is in some way linked to oxidation and its release of free radicals, the exact process still needs to be worked out. Dr. Abraham Spector, professor of ophthalmic biochemistry at Columbia University College of Physicians and Surgeons, is one of the leaders in research in human cataracts. He has found evidence of free radicals such as hydrogen peroxide in the aqueous fluid that surrounds and nourishes the lens. This peroxide, identical to the bottled kind available at your local pharmacy, is toxic to the lens and likely to be a cause for loss of transparency and cataract formation. Dr. Kailash Bhuyan, a leading cataract researcher at New York's Mount Sinai Hospital, is convinced that oxidation of the lipid portion of cells in the lens eventually leads to damage and cataract formation. Bhuyan has shown in experimental cataract models and in human cataracts that free radicals are found in excessive amounts and are improperly neutralized.

Evidence for the harmful effects of oxidation in cataract formation includes the finding of cataracts in patients exposed to high oxygen levels, the finding of oxidized lens protein in aged and cataractous lenses, and the protective effect of the antioxidant BHF (commonly added to foods to prevent spoilage) in preventing cataracts in laboratory animals.

I mention all of this not just to round out your education in advanced biochemistry but to prepare you for the good news. Once scientists and doctors know what causes a disorder, prevention and cure can follow. With cataracts, surgery is still the only cure, but for the first time ever, prevention is a definite possibility. If oxidation is a cause of cataracts, blocking oxidation of lens protein will prevent them. Fortunately, we all have enzymes and chemicals in our eyes and throughout our body that act as antioxidants and neutralize the harmful effects of free radicals and oxidation. These chemicals are similar to the ones that give antirust paint its special properties. Since the "antirust" chemicals in our own lenses are not always successful in blocking cataract formation, due to their very low concentration, antioxidant vitamins such as Vitamin E in our diet may prevent us from developing cataracts. Studies so far are very promising. We will return to cataract prevention later on in Chapter 12. We will also discuss the importance of wearing sunglasses that block ultraviolet light.

Other Causes

Although the normal aging process accounts, probably through oxidative stress, for the majority of cataracts in the general population, diabetes plays a significant role in cataract formation in the diabetic population. About 10 to 15 percent of patients with cataracts also suffer from diabetes, a disorder characterized by elevated blood sugar levels. Researchers in the field of diabetes and cataracts are close to a real understanding of the true cause of cataracts—and possible medical, rather than surgical, treatment. The longer the duration of diabetes, especially in females, the more likely the chance of developing a cataract. Poor control of blood sugar as well as long duration of diabetes may play a role in cataract development. This fact ought to provide further incentive for diabetic patients to be more careful about diet, medication, and medical checkups.

Solid evidence for the link between cataracts and diabetes is based on a study of nearly five thousand people in the area of Framingham, Massachusetts, published in the *American Journal of Ophthalmology* in 1981. The study showed that if you have diabetes and are under age seventy, you have a 30 to 40 percent greater chance of having a cataract than another person without diabetes the same age. Past age seventy, the diabetes and age factors are about equal, so diabetics and nondiabetics have an equal chance of developing a cataract.

Juvenile diabetics—patients who develop diabetes at an early age, usually under age thirty—tend to have wider fluctuations in blood sugar than patients with adult-onset diabetes, and it is the wide variation in blood sugar that is thought to cause swelling of the lens in the eye, loss of transparency, and a resultant cataract. In that terrifying era before Frederick Banting and Charles Best discovered insulin as the treatment for diabetes in 1922, it was not uncommon for a juvenile diabetic to develop a sudden, blinding cloudiness of the lens, called a *sugar cataract*, brought on by a blood sugar level wildly out of control. Fortunately, this type of cataract is very rare today.

What finally emerged in the early 1980s, largely from studies by cataract researchers Dr. Jin Kinoshita and Dr. Leo T. Chylack of Boston, Massachusetts, is that too much sugar in the blood actually causes cataracts. This was quite a significant discovery, and it advanced our knowledge of cataracts a great deal. Three sugars were studied, two of which were found to have a direct effect on human cataract formation. The first sugar, glucose, is present in ordinary table sugar; the second, galactose, is found in milk and dairy products. These sugars, known as aldose sugars, dissolve into the lens of the diabetic and are converted into substances that cause the lens to swell rapidly with the aqueous fluid surrounding it, like a dry sponge suddenly immersed in water. This bloating of the lens with fluid upsets the delicate balance that keeps it clear, resulting in a dense cataract. The culprit in all this seems to be an innocent-appearing enzyme, aldose reductase, which is triggered by high levels of sugar in the eye and which converts the aldose sugars to a form that can cause cataracts.

Several substances have been developed that can block sugar cataract formation in laboratory animals, and an exhaustive search is underway for a means to block cataract formation in humans with diabetes. Several pharmaceutical companies are trying to develop safe drugs that can block aldose reductase, since this enzyme definitely seems responsible for the formation of sugar cataracts. Perhaps this research eventually will lead to medical rather than surgical treatment of senile cataracts as well.

Let me hasten to add that with modern eye care, including cataract and laser surgery, the vast majority of diabetic patients will maintain good vision their whole lives. For patients with severe diabetic eye disease, the prognosis has never been better for maintaining good vision. Good control of your diabetes and regular visits to your ophthalmologist will help ensure that you remain in the vast majority.

The stimulus for all this work on glucose, diabetes, and sugar cataracts actually came from the study of infants with *galactosemia*, a rare disease that affects about one out of every 18,000 newborns. Galactosemia results in severe malnutrition for the baby no matter how much milk he or she drinks. The reason for the seeming paradox of malnutrition in the face of plenty is the lack of an enzyme that enables the baby to digest galactose, a component of the principal sugar in milk, lactose. Without this enzyme the otherwise healthy baby cannot get proper nourishment, and if the disease is not recognized quickly the baby will die in one or two months.

One of the effects of the undigested galactose in the newborn is that it is converted by aldose reductase to a substance that accumulates in the lens in very high amounts. In over 75 percent of cases it causes a severe cataract. The ophthalmologist's role is crucial, because the dense, white cataracts are often the first sign of this otherwise fatal disease. Treatment is simple—take the baby off all milk products and substitute soy milk, which lacks the milk sugar galactose. If recognized before four weeks of age, the prognosis is excellent: The cataract will disappear and the baby's health will return. The crucial role of the ophthalmologist in galactosemia is one of the many ways ophthalmologists can diagnose a general disease from symptoms and signs that seem to involve only the eye.

Although a very small segment of the population is directly affected by the missing galactose sugar enzyme, a much greater segment, children and adults alike, have milder, less serious forms of milk intolerance that may reflect a partial loss of the same enzyme. One of the questions I always ask a young person with cataracts is "How do you like milk?" If the answer is "I like it, but my stomach doesn't," I think of the galactose enzyme. There is no hard evidence for a link between senile cataracts and milk intolerance, but there certainly is evidence for it in juvenile cataracts. The diagnosis is made by several simple blood and urine tests, which should be done on all babies and children with cataracts.

Babies without any milk intolerance at all can still be born with cataracts in one or even both eyes. This occurs in about one out of every 3,000 to 4,000 births. These congenital cataracts can be small localized opacities in the lens that do not interfere with vision, or can involve total clouding of the entire lens with resulting blindness. We now recognize that if the baby is to regain useful vision in the eye with the cataract, surgery *must* be performed within the first few months of life. You have only to imagine operating on cataracts in a two-month-old to appreciate the wonders of microsurgery.

A congenital cataract is usually discovered by a parent, who notices a white pupil in the baby's eye instead of the normally black one. There are many causes of congenital cataracts; the common denominator is something that interferes with the normal development of the lens in the fetus. Medications taken by the mother during pregnancy can adversely affect the developing eye, especially cortisone-type drugs and certain tranquilizers. Premature babies are more apt to have a congenital cataract than full-term babies. German measles or rubella infection in the mother, especially during the last part of the first three months of pregnancy, can seriously affect the developing eye, causing congenital cataracts in the majority of cases. Fortunately, the widespread use of vaccines to prevent German measles have made congenital cataracts less common.

Congenital cataracts represent not only a technical challenge—the surgery itself—but a rehabilitative one. If the baby is to regain useful vision, the eye must start to see almost immediately after surgery. This could be accomplished by thick cataract glasses, by a contact lens, or in some cases by an intraocular lens implant, as is invariably used in adults. If good vision is not restored early after cataract surgery, the eye will become "lazy" and vision will be poor, despite an otherwise successful operation.

Of course, the majority of children pass through infancy without galactose sugar or congenital cataracts. But they are vulnerable to a more common cataract—the traumatic cataract. This type of cataract develops from an injury to the eye, either one in which an object penetrates the eye and touches the delicate clear lens, or one that jars the lens enough to damage it. As an ophthalmologist I hate July Fourth with its parades and firecrackers. Out of those thousands of children patriotically and frantically waving their flags, dueling with their brothers and sisters, and running back and forth, some will fall. We can hope that at worst the child will scratch his or her arm, not the eye, but I have seen enough eye injuries to shudder at the thought of another parade. Most eye injuries are not serious, but the exception to the rule does happen all too frequently. I often hear my children muttering "eccentric" under their breath when I caution them about walking about carrying scissors, pencils, or anything with an end that even faintly resembles a point. Never, *ever*, let children play with anything with a pointed end.

Many other causes of cataracts are quite rare and even sometimes bizarre. Glass blowers are prone to cataracts, apparently from constant exposure to intense heat. Electrical workers may develop cataracts from electric shock, and patients who undergo electroconvulsive shock treatments for various psychiatric disorders may develop cataracts. Even other eye diseases such as iritis, an inflammation of the iris, can lead to cataracts. Cataracts that result from eye disease are called *secondary cataracts*.

There is some evidence, so far inconclusive, that malnutrition may play a role in causing cataracts. Malnutrition is often a combination of protein, vitamin, and mineral deficiencies, and it is not clear which if any of these factors is responsible should a cataract develop.

A fascinating study was performed in 1982 by Dr. Harold Skalka, chairman of the department of ophthalmology at the University of Alabama School of Medicine. He examined 173 older people and found that one-third of them had evidence of riboflavin, or Vitamin B_2, deficiency. This was nothing new, as previous surveys of nutrition in the older age group of the United States had found the same thing. However, what was interesting was that of the 173 people studied, 16 of them, or about 10 percent, had an absolutely clear lens in each eye with no trace of a cataract. These 16 people not only showed no Vitamin B_2 deficiency but had higher levels of Vitamin B_2 than even healthy young adults. When these 16 adults with no evidence of a cataract were matched with 53 adults with cataracts, the main difference was in the level of Vitamin B_2. This finding was quite significant. It does not mean, however, that everyone over sixty-five should immediately run to the nearest Vitamin B_2 supplier, for this is only one small study.

Most other studies evaluating the relationship between nutrition and cataracts in the United States have been less conclusive. In 1988 Dr. Leo Chylack and colleagues studied 77 patients with cataracts and 35 similar patients without cataracts. The nutritional status for all patients was determined by measuring blood levels of various vitamins and nutrients. Vitamin D and carotenoids, precursors of Vitamin A, seemed to offer some protection against developing cataracts. Other vitamins, including Vitamin C and Vitamin E, as well as the minerals copper, magnesium, and zinc, did not seem to offer any protection against cataract formation. Although no useful conclusions for the role of nutrition in cataract formation could be drawn from this study, many other more recent studies do tend to support a protective effect for certain vitamins and minerals, as we shall see in Chapter 12.

If the role for nutrition in cataract formation in the United States is still unclear, it is quite convincing in third world and underdeveloped countries. More specifically, life-threatening diarrhea and dehydration have been definitely implicated in causing cataracts, and in India alone, 1.5 million new cases of blindness each year are attributable to severe diarrhea. Of the 13 million people each year blind from cataract in developing countries, there are almost 4 million newly blind from cataracts in India alone. To treat existing patients in India and keep up with new ones, 5 million cataract operations would need to be performed each year. Since such countries have nowhere near enough ophthalmologists to cope with the problem, the importance of nutrition and prevention of dehydration and diarrhea in the third world cannot be overemphasized.

Although low levels of calcium can also lead to cataracts, the cause is usually not poor nutrition or lack of calcium in our diet, but improper working of four tiny glands in the neck, the parathyroid glands. These glands regulate the level of calcium in our blood. Their malfunction, if untreated, will cause low blood calcium and cataracts, regardless of how much calcium we get in our diet.

Cataracts are fairly common in individuals who must take continuous doses of cortisone for prolonged periods of time. Several illnesses, such as arthritis, asthma, gastrointestinal disorders, and autoimmune-type diseases such as lupus, are often best treated by cortisone, which puts the patient in an unfortunate dilemma. The medication is needed to control the illness, but cataracts may ensue. Prednisone and other cortisone preparations cause a specific type of opacification of the back part of the lens just under the capsule. This posterior subcapsular cataract is quite characteristic of prolonged cortisone use and takes years and years to develop. In general, the smaller the dose and the shorter the course of cortisone medication, the less chance you have of developing a cataract. There is a wide range of susceptibility to cataract formation, and in some individuals even small doses over a relatively short period of time can result in a cataract. You and your doctor must weigh the risks and benefits of cortisone use in treating your illness. If you do need to take cortisone for a long period of time, make sure to see your ophthalmologist at least once or twice a year. The success rate for cataract removal is the same, whether your cataract was caused by cortisone use or malnutrition or age. But you should ensure that your general dietary habits are optimum, not only for Vitamin B_2 but for all vitamins and minerals.

In the past, glaucoma sufferers had a similar dilemma. It was known for some time that patients who suffer from glaucoma, an eye disease in which the pressure in the eye is higher than normal, tend to get cataracts more frequently than do the general population. In the early days of glaucoma therapy, most patients used eyedrops called miotics, such as phospholine iodide, to lower the eye pressure and thus prevent damage to the eye and preserve sight. However, these same glaucoma drops probably caused tens of thousands of cataracts in unsuspecting glaucoma patients. The drops continuously regulated the pressure in the eye; they acted like a spigot in a water barrel, constantly letting enough fluid out to avoid a buildup of pressure. With the advent of newer antiglaucoma drops, patients were able to switch from the offending eyedrop to others that play no role in cataract formation. Thus one source of cataracts has been eliminated. Should a patient with glaucoma develop a cataract, surgery can successfully remove it, as we will soon discuss.

The latest possible cause of cataracts in an increasingly

long list is cigarette smoking. According to two studies published in August 1992 in the *Journal of the American Medical Association (JAMA)*, cigarette smokers have a significantly higher risk of developing cataracts than nonsmokers. The two studies from the Harvard Medical School, one by Dr. William Christen on over 17,000 American male physicians, and another by Dr. Susan Hankinson on 69,000 female nurses, showed that cigarette smokers more than doubled their risk of developing cataracts. In referring to the study, Dr. Sheila West, an ophthalmologist at Baltimore's Johns Hopkins Hospital, concluded that smoking is responsible for approximately 20 percent of cataracts in the U.S. population. The many maladies associated with smoking continue to grow in number.

5

How to Choose an Ophthalmologist

Most people have a family medical doctor who is consulted for checkups and for treatment of colds, flu, stomach upsets, and more serious illnesses, such as hypertension and heart disease, as well as a dentist for preventive checkups and dental care. Many women have a gynecologist whom they see regularly for a variety of problems and for the all-important annual pap smear. People ordinarily do not have a neurosurgeon, proctologist, or radiologist; these highly specialized doctors generally are consulted only on referral by a family medical doctor who suspects a problem needing further diagnosis and treatment. Though also highly specialized, the ophthalmologist is certainly high on the list of doctors most people will see with some regularity throughout their lives. In addition to performing eye surgery, ophthalmologists treat many different eye conditions, including conjunctivitis (pinkeye) and glaucoma, and also prescribe eyeglasses. Many patients see an optometrist rather than an ophthalmologist for their eye care, and will often go to yet a third professional, the optician, to purchase eyeglasses. What is the difference?

An *optometrist* is a doctor of optometry (O.D. instead of the ophthalmologist's M.D.) and is *not* a physician. Optometrists have been through college and four years of optometry school where they studied a variety of subjects pertaining to the mechanism and diagnosis of eye disease. During their training optometrists also develop skills in refracting the eye—that is, determining the need for glasses and giving a suitable prescription. They also thoroughly study the fitting, formulation, and sale of eyeglasses and contact lenses.

Optometrists who are skilled in refractions, contact lenses, and dispensing of glasses as well as diagnosing common eye problems perform a valuable service for their patients. Many patients I see were first told of cataracts or glaucoma by their local optometrist, who then rightly advised the patient to seek the care of an ophthalmologist.

An *ophthalmologist* is first a physician, a medical doctor, just as a neurosurgeon or general practitioner is a physician. The ophthalmologist has been through college, four years of medical school, one year of internship, and at least three years of specialized residency training in diseases and surgery of the eye. Some ophthalmologists then go on to subspecialize. This means one or two more years of training in just one type of eye disease. A corneal surgeon who performs corneal transplants or a retinal surgeon who only does surgery for detached retinas are two examples of such subspecialization.

Cataract surgeons are usually general ophthalmologists who develop their skills during their three or more years of residency training and enter private or hospital practice after their training is completed. They learn new techniques in courses given throughout the country or by visiting and operating with experts in the field. Although general ophthalmologists will also do glaucoma, cornea, and retina surgery, they spend most of their operating time doing cataract surgery. While this may seem repetitious and unstimulating, most of the joy in any field of ophthalmic surgery comes from fairly specialized, exacting surgery done week after week.

Opticians, the third group in the eye-care triumvirate, are trained in taking the eyeglass prescription you get from the doctor, helping you select a suitable frame, and grinding and formulating lenses to make a pair of spectacles. In some states, such as New York, opticians can also fit and dispense contact lenses in much the same way as do ophthalmologists or optometrists. They are not trained or licensed to examine the eye, only to make the glasses or contact lenses.

If you suspect a cataract as the source of your eye trouble or if you suspect your problem is something other than can be cured with glasses, you should be under the care of an ophthalmologist. Through medical school and internship he or she has built up a foundation of knowledge and an understanding of how diseases affect the human body, how they progress, how symptoms can be narrowed down to one diagnosis when they initially seem to represent ten or twenty. All this knowledge becomes so ingrained that much of it is subconscious and forms the basis of the most precious skill a physician can possess—judgment. Diagnoses can now be made by computers, and surgical techniques can be taught to many technicians, but judgment is a decision-making ability that is largely based on subconscious, often innate, qualities that are difficult to learn. Judgment means being able to tell which patient with a headache needs the aspirin and which needs the neurosurgeon. Judgment means knowing which patient is truly unhappy with his eyesight and needs cataract surgery, and which patient can still function well enough to delay surgery and merely needs reassurance and encouragement.

How do you go about finding an ophthalmologist, or any physician for that matter, with diagnostic acumen, surgical skill, impeccable character, good judgment, and warm personality? Assuming that you are successful in your search, what happens if you do not like him or her, if there is no "chemistry" between you? It would be wonderful to find in that gifted eye surgeon someone you also like, can talk to, and can call at two in the morning without quaking with fear, should there be a problem. Confidence and trust are extremely important in a good relationship between patient and doctor, for without this you may become disenchanted with the doctor in spite of what may be a technically perfect surgical result.

Following are six ways to find an ophthalmologist, listed in order of preference. We will examine each method in detail, as each has its benefits and drawbacks.

1. Stay with the one you have.
2. Ask your family doctor.
3. Ask the chief resident of ophthalmology at a major hospital.
4. Ask a friend or relative.
5. Consult the phone book.
6. Call the local medical society.

Staying with your Current Ophthalmologist

If you are already under the care of an ophthalmologist you like and have faith in, you are one step ahead and need go no further in selecting an eye surgeon. This is probably the most ideal situation. The vast majority of ophthalmologists throughout the country are extremely well trained in cataract surgery and will do an excellent job. After reading this book you will understand the different types of cataract surgery and will be better able to match your goals with those of your eye doctor.

Referral from the Family Doctor

A referral from your family doctor is one of the best means available for choosing an ophthalmologist, but it is not foolproof. Let's say you are seventy years old and have been seeing your medical doctor for five or ten years. You may have initially consulted him or her for a specific problem such as high blood pressure or flu or may have needed only a checkup. Over the years you've consulted the doctor for various problems. You have always been quite pleased with his treatment and judgment and have developed confidence and trust in him, not only as a physician but as a friend. What better way to locate his ophthalmologic counterpart than to ask him? He will naturally want you to have the best care and would most likely feel personally responsible for his choice of an eye doctor. He should recommend the person he thinks is best qualified to remove your cataract, the ophthalmologist he would use for his own family should cataract surgery be needed. But will he? Will he truly know the best-qualified eye doctor? The answer is usually yes, but sometimes no.

Doctors do not belong to any exclusive medical club where members are privy to the strengths and weaknesses of everyone else and all band together secretly to exchange vows of silence. If I were to need a doctor to fix a broken hip or do open-heart surgery, I would have somewhat of a head start over the average patient in my search for the ideal doctor, but I would still need to get recommendations and then decide. In the end, I would probably have an easier, quicker, and more fruitful search than you, but it would still require a search and a decision. For most patients, the help of a trusted family physician will make your decision easier. Doctors do tend to recommend their friends and colleagues, but friendship and loyalty should be secondary to recommending someone most suitable for your needs.

If your medical doctor has had your trust and faith over the years, the specialists he or she uses will merit this same relationship. Since you are probably not the first patient she's had to refer to an ophthalmologist for cataract surgery, she will have formed an opinion over the years about which ophthalmologists her patients seem to do best with, and she will have developed confidence in their ability. She should be able to match your personality against the ophthalmologist to whom you will be referred. Most likely she will refer you to someone on the staff of the same hospital as she, so that should the need arise, she will be available to see you in the hospital. You might ask your family doctor if she's had many patients who have used this ophthalmologist for cataract surgery and perhaps speak to one or two of them about their experience. This is much more sensible than asking your ophthalmologist for the names of several patients on whom he's operated, as this selection will naturally be biased.

Referral from a Chief Resident

The second means of finding an ophthalmologist to take care of your cataracts is often the best, but it too is by no means foolproof and it can often be the most difficult. Call the eye clinic at a nearby large medical center, preferably a teaching hospital, and request to speak to the chief resident in ophthalmology. You will usually be put through to an ophthalmology resident who is almost finished with his training. This resident should be able to give an objective recommendation for two or three ophthalmologists he feels are especially skilled in cataract surgery. More than likely he will have operated with these ophthalmologists, assisting them and in turn having them assist him. He should have formed an opinion about their capabilities and be in a good position to provide several names. Before seeking a recommendation, you should try to find out whether you are a good candidate for the relatively new small-incision surgery. One ophthalmologist may be more experienced in this type of surgery while another may be better suited for the more standard type of cataract surgery. We will discuss the different types of cataract surgery in Chapter 7.

By finding an ophthalmologist through this sort of referral, you may overlook many highly skilled eye surgeons who are so busy in private practice that they do not have time to teach in a hospital. Recommendations from two or three different sources would be helpful.

Lay Recommendation

A third way to find an ophthalmologist is through a recommendation from a friend, relative, or neighbor. This may be a blessing or a calamity, and the odds may be fifty-fifty. The key is the person from whom you are getting the recommendation. Is the person discriminating and reliable? Was that great internist your cousin recommended the type of doctor you would want in an ophthalmologist? Does your cousin tell you the good as well as the bad, or is she the type who automatically knows only "the best"—the best Italian restaurant, the best accountant, the best ophthalmologist? Even with the best of intentions, a visit to an eye doctor enthusiastically recommended by a friend or relative may leave you unimpressed. There are several reasons for this: Your son or daughter may have seen an eye doctor for reasons other than a cataract, such as contact lenses or glaucoma, and the doctor may be better for those problems than for cataracts and cataract surgery. Perhaps the doctor does not use the newer methods of cataract surgery or does not do small-incision surgery. She may not be the right surgeon for you, then. It is therefore a good idea to ask your referral source how he or she got the doctor's name. Perhaps two or three other people you know have used that doctor and can attest to her skill.

Phone Book

Flipping through the "Physicians" section of the phone book and selecting the ophthalmologist whose location is the most convenient is a poor way to select someone to examine your eyes and perhaps operate on them. By doing so, it is purely a matter of luck if you do select someone you like and trust to advise you on surgery and to remove your cataracts. What you think may be a simple eyeglass problem may be more serious, so ophthalmologists or any doctor, for that matter, should be selected carefully. The Yellow Pages is a terrific way to find a neighborhood pharmacy or liquor store, but it is not the recommended way to locate a physician. The size of the advertisement has no bearing on the doctor's competence.

A listing of physicians and surgeons grouped by specialty is, however, a great help when you are in a strange city and need an ophthalmologist, since the phone book may be your only source for doctors. At least it is a starting point in locating a physician when other avenues are unavailable.

If you do need to locate an ophthalmologist through the phone book, you should ask several questions on the phone. No staff member in an office should hesitate to supply this information.

Is the doctor board certified? While having board certification does not necessarily indicate any level of surgical skill, it is some measure of the level of knowledge, since board certification requires passing a series of oral and written examinations after residency training is completed. Board certification should be a minimum standard of excellence.

From what medical school did the doctor graduate? Although I know many excellent physicians who are graduates of a foreign medical school, other things being equal, it is better to see a graduate of an American medical school, since the clinical training is often superior.

With what hospital is the doctor affiliated? Most large cities have teaching hospitals where medical students, interns, and residents learn and work and do research as well as teach. Physicians exposed to this educational milieu are often more stimulated than are their counterparts in nonteaching hospitals to keep up with advances in their fields. If you are not familiar with the hospital affiliation of the ophthalmologist, ask if it is a teaching hospital and whether it has a residency program in ophthalmology. The academic atmosphere of the hospital, clinical skills of the physicians, and general patient care tend to be above average at teaching hospitals.

If you are planning a move to a strange city, ask your current eye doctor to recommend an ophthalmologist well versed in cataracts and cataract surgery. He may know someone to whom he can refer you, even if you are moving thousands of miles away. If he does not know someone in the vicinity of your proposed move, he can consult the *Directory of the American Academy of Ophthalmology*, which list ophthalmologists throughout the country, grouped by state and city. The books give brief biographies of the physicians, including medical school, board certification, and subspecialty, if any. This is quite a bit better than taking potluck with the Yellow Pages.

Referral from a Local Medical Society

Well-meaning consumer groups often tout checking with the referral service of your local medical society as a good recommendation for a doctor. However, to get listed in the referral service for his or her specialty, or *any* subspecialty in which the doctor feels qualified, the doctor usually need only join the society and pay dues. The medical society makes no attempt to verify the qualifications of its members, nor does it conduct any follow-up with patients referred to the doctors. If you call the local medical society for a referral to an ophthalmologist, say, you will receive the names of several who feel qualified in the area of your concern and who practice in your vicinity. Not only is this information often inaccurate, it can also give you a false sense of security. A busy, successful ophthalmologist may not encourage the few extra referrals from the medical society and may not be listed in the service at all. Although many excellent and highly competent doctors are listed, getting a doctor through such a listing is little better than using a phone book. Any reputable medical society should eliminate referrals to doctors found to be less than highly qualified or ethical, but with the current system patients have no way of knowing anything about the skills of the doctors.

There are several simple ways of rectifying the system of referrals from the medical society. The society should run a check on the physicians who want to be on the referral service by consulting with the chairpeople of the department in which the physicians trained. Their quali-fications can be checked against their application. The referral service would then have some confidence in these doctors' capabilities. The medical society should also send follow-up cards to patients it refers for help in future refer-rals. Until more quality assurance is built into the system, it is foolhardy to rely on the medical society for locating an ophthalmologist who performs cataract surgery, or in-deed for finding any physician.

The Second Opinion

You may often hear of the advisability of obtaining a second opinion, either to help resolve a doubtful diagnosis or treatment plan or to confirm what was said by your own doctor. In the past, many insurance companies required a second opinion for cataract and other types of "elective" surgery in a misguided effort to reduce "unnecessary" surgery. Most insurance companies have recently reviewed the need for a second opinion in cataract cases, since their own statistics show the second opinion to agree with the first over 95 percent of the time. The Office of the U.S. Inspector General found that the first opinion in cataract surgery consultations was correct 98 percent of the time, the highest such rate in any surgical subspecialty. According to a 1990 U.S. Health and Human Services Department review of 500,000 cataract operations paid for by Medicare, the U.S. paid an independent review organization $13.3 million to save $1.4 million in "possibly unnecessary surgery."[1] The second opinion is less than cost-effective, but it is still required by some insurance companies.

A second opinion may be appropriate if you are not comfortable with your current ophthalmologist; however, when it comes to cataract surgery, only you know how much your vision is bothering you and how much trouble you are having at work or in your daily activities. **The most important second opinion is really your own.** After

[1] *Wall Street Journal*, July 28, 1992.

reading this book you should be able to understand cataracts better and to talk to your ophthalmologist more confidently about the options of cataract surgery, judging whether his or her approach and recommendations agree with your own. You can make as intelligent and informed a judgment as possible about the person who will operate on your eye. Your second opinion will be almost as valuable as the first opinion given by your ophthalmologist, whose advice and guidance, in light of your newly found knowledge, will have more meaning and ensure as much as possible a successful outcome.

6

The Eye Examination

Have you ever wondered about all those instruments and gadgets your eye doctor uses? During your eye examination you may be bombarded with bright lights, dim lights, white lights, red lights, green lights, blue lights, eyedrops, lenses on the eye, and lenses in front of the eye. Although I try to explain each step of my examination to my patients, I know that it is almost impossible to come away from the eye examination knowing just what your ophthalmologist did to arrive at the decision to operate on your cataract. In order to share in the decision to have surgery, you must understand what is done in the eye examination. This chapter explains the purpose, scope, and procedures of the eye examination. Once you understand that, you will be a better patient. You will be better able to explain to your ophthalmologist what is bothering you and, therefore, more important, your doctor will be able to help you more effectively and efficiently.

The eye examination consists of five main parts:

1. History
2. Visual acuity and refraction
3. External examination
4. Slit-lamp examination
5. Retina examination

History

Introductions and social amenities concluded, you are in the examining chair. Your eye doctor asks, "What is the trouble?" Your answer will probably be something like "My vision is getting worse. I have more and more trouble reading and even need a magnifying glass for small print." Or, "I can't recognize bus signs or people in the street." "I can't watch TV." "I can't do my normal work any more."

Whatever your actual answer, the basic problem that prompted your examination is vision. It is not pain, tearing, discharge, or itching, which are common eye symptoms unrelated to cataracts. It is vision. A most important part of the history comes next. "Was this a gradual loss of vision or was it sudden?" Cataracts usually grow slowly, and the accompanying visual loss is likewise slowly progressive. Sudden visual loss should alert the ophthalmologist to causes other than cataracts, such as a hemorrhage in the retina or a detached retina. Hardening of the arteries or arteriosclerosis can result in insufficient blood flow to the optic nerve causing sudden loss of vision. Although sudden loss of vision in one eye speaks against a cataract, the loss of vision may indeed come from that, especially if the cataract is in your nondominant eye. As mentioned earlier, you may be surprisingly unaware of the cataract for years. When you suddenly notice it, you may be in a state of panic and will hurriedly call your eye doctor. The visual loss was gradual, but your awareness was sudden.

Your ophthalmologist will also ask you about pain. A cataract is almost always painless. The presence of pain may mean an inflammation of the eye called uveitis, or an increase of pressure in the eye, glaucoma. Loss of vision accompanied by pain is unlikely to be due to cataracts but can be serious, and you should contact your ophthalmologist immediately.

You will also be asked about your general health, since it can affect your eyes. Diabetes or high blood pressure can alter vision by adversely affecting the retina. It is important to differentiate between cataracts and retina trouble as a cause for poor eyesight. Removing a cataract from an eye with a retina seriously weakened by diabetes may not significantly improve vision.

Visual Acuity and Refraction

After the history is taken, your eye doctor will have you read the eye chart to determine the level of acuity, or sight, in each eye. Each eye is assigned the level of vision corresponding to the lowest line of the eye chart or the smallest letters that can be read by that eye, such as 20/40, 20/70, or 20/200. If one of your eyes can see only the biggest figure on the chart, such as the "big E," the vision for that eye is listed as 20/400. If your other eye sees 20/20, you, as a whole, with both eyes open, will still see 20/20, but your "bad eye" will contribute only 20/400, a small amount, to your total vision. If one eye cannot even see 20/400 but can count how many fingers your eye doctor holds up, the vision is called "count fingers." If the separated fingers cannot even be discerned but the hand can be seen vaguely to move, the vision is known as hand motion. The next worse vision is light perception, or LP, when only the presence or absence of light can be noticed. The worst vision is NLP, or no light perception, when even the strongest light possible is the same as total darkness. To an ophthalmologist, NLP is the equivalent of total blindness. An increasingly dense cataract will naturally give increasingly poor vision, but no cataract can be so severe as to block out light completely.

After your vision is checked, the ophthalmologist will then perform a refraction—trying different lenses to see which combination will give the best corrected vision in each eye. As you look at certain letters on the eye chart, the eye doctor will try different lenses in front of each eye, and you will be asked to make a choice: "Which is better, lens 1, or lens 2?" This often drives patients frantic, since it seems equivalent to a test in grade school. But unlike grade school, there is no right or wrong answer. Just pick whichever lens makes the letters look clearer and sharper.

The refraction may be performed with a trial frame, a heavy metal frame with slots for lenses, or with a device called a phoroptor. The phoroptor resembles a giant butterfly and contains hundreds of lenses that can be flipped in front of each eye at the turn of a dial. It is usually suspended from a stand or attached to the wall and is moved in front of your eyes at the start of the refraction. Many ophthalmologists have computerized instruments that can do the refraction automatically in a few seconds. A technician or assistant usually performs the automated refraction, but in the end your eye doctor will still badger you with "Which is better, one or two?" After the best vision for distance is determined, other lenses will be placed over your distance prescription to achieve the best vision for reading. There may be a big discrepancy between your far and near acuity, since cataracts may blur vision differently at distance and near. The level of your vision is one of the best indications of the health of your eye and the severity of your cataract, and is as basic to your eye health as your blood pressure is to your general health.

External Examination

The third part of the eye examination, the external examination, is done with a small flashlight called a penlight. The doctor will look at your eyelids and pupils, and check the eye muscles and eye position. The lids are often prone to a chronic inflammation called blepharitis, usually associated with seborrhea (oiliness of the skin) and dandruff of the scalp and eyelashes. If significant blepharitis is present during cataract surgery, there may be an increased chance of infection. Your doctor will advise you on treatment, which usually consists of hot compresses and cleaning of the lids with a cotton swab and baby shampoo or eyelid cleaner followed by antibiotic ointment.

Your eyelid position will also be checked, since a slight droop of one lid or a slight asymmetry of the lids is fairly common and should be noted prior to any eye surgery. The upper lid may tend to droop slightly after cataract surgery, and while this situation is usually temporary, a droopy lid can be permanent. To check the pupils, the doctor will shine the penlight into each eye, alternating the light from one eye to the other. Each pupil should equally and briskly constrict to light. An abnormal pupil may indicate another problem with the eye besides a cataract. A cataract, no matter how dense, will not affect the working of the pupils.

Next, the doctor will examine the soundness of the six eye muscles. He or she will ask you to follow an object up, down, left, and right. The eyes should be perfectly aligned and work as a pair and not be crossed or drifting apart or drifting up or down. A cataract in one eye, present for years and years, depriving that eye of good vision, may cause the eye to drift out of alignment, usually outward— that is, away from your nose. This would normally cause double vision, but if the cataract blocks the vision in one eye, you may not notice the blurred double image until vision is restored by cataract surgery. It is important to predict if this may happen, because double vision can be as annoying as was the original cataract. Fortunately, the double vision will usually clear up spontaneously after cataract surgery, once the eyes start working together.

Slit-Lamp Examination

The slit-lamp examination, the fourth step in the eye examination, enables your ophthalmologist to examine your cataract to determine how "ripe," or mature, it is. Another name for the slit lamp is a biomicroscope, a very apt description because it does give a magnified, microscopic view of the front parts of the eye—cornea, iris, and lens— collectively called the anterior segment of the eye. The slit lamp is wheeled into place in front of you, and you rest your chin on the chin rest and your forehead against a headrest. Your doctor will look through two eyepieces that look like binoculars and focus a vertical slit beam of light onto your cataract. With the room lights off and the room quiet, you may think you've wandered onto the set of *Star Wars*. By changing the focus and the angle of the slit of light, the doctor can examine all parts of your cataract completely. In this way, he or she can decide how dense the cataract is and what type of cataract surgery will be best for you.

The slit beam of light will also be used to examine your cornea carefully for signs of weakness. The back part of the cornea is slightly weakened or stressed during cataract surgery. The stress can cause slight temporary clouding of the cornea, sometimes persisting for days or weeks or rarely permanently after surgery. Your eye doctor will make sure your cornea is healthy enough to withstand the slight stress of cataract surgery. The presence of Fuch's dystrophy, a weakness of the endothelium (the back part of the cornea) can be easily diagnosed during the slit-lamp examination and will alert your doctor to the possibility that a cloudy cornea after surgery may be likely. Although a cloudy cornea usually clears after cataract surgery, a severely compromised cornea may not, necessitating a corneal transplant in the future.

Dry eyes, a condition almost as common as cataracts in people as they age, are due to decreased production of tears from glands under the upper and lower lids. These tears are produced twenty-four hours a day and lubricate the eye, as opposed to the tears from crying or peeling onions, which are produced only when the eye is stimulated or irritated. Since dry eyes can get drier after cataract surgery, possibly due to the strong light from the microscope shining on your eye as the doctor operates, it is important that dry eye syndrome be diagnosed prior to surgery so that you can receive artificial teardrops to keep the eye moist and clear after surgery. A dry and lackluster cornea can delay recovery of vision in an otherwise perfectly performed cataract operation. Artificial teardrops and ointments are usually effective in restoring moisture to the eye.

Attached to the slit lamp is a tonometer, a probelike device for measuring the intraocular pressure (the pressure inside your eye). An anesthetic drop is instilled in each eye and a piece of paper impregnated with fluorescein, an orange dye, is painlessly touched to the inside of each lower lid. Some of the dye dissolves in your tears and coats the cornea. The doctor changes the white beam of light to a blue light by flipping a lever on the slit-lamp arm and then slowly moves the tonometer probe toward your eye.

Looking through the slit lamp, your ophthalmologist will see a fluorescent pattern as the probe gently touches your cornea. The force needed to make this pattern is equal to the intraocular pressure. The test is painless and simple and need not cause any anxiety. The normal intraocular pressure is usually between 14 and 21 millimeters of mercury, the same unit of measure as in blood pressure; a reading over twenty-one may indicate the presence of glaucoma. Since cataract surgery is safer when the eye pressure is normal or even below normal, it is extremely important for your doctor to measure your eye pressure before your operation.

You will also undergo a test called gonioscopy. In this test, the doctor checks the anterior chamber angle (the angle the cornea makes with the iris) with a mirrored lens called a gonioscope. It is through this angle that fluid drains out of the eye; when this drainage gets blocked, the pressure will rise and glaucoma may ensue.

It is important that your doctor do this test, for several reasons. The angle should be very wide open, rather than narrow or closed. If the angle is very narrow, dilating drops can further narrow it and block fluid from leaving the eye, causing a rapid rise in intraocular pressure and acute glaucoma. Just prior to cataract surgery the pupil needs to be very dilated. (Eyedrops are used to accomplish this.) If this dilation causes a severe rise in intraocular pressure, complications may result during the surgery.

Another reason that your doctor must check the anterior chamber angle with the gonioscope is that if an anterior chamber implant will be placed it must fit snugly into this angle. (We examine this implant closely in Chapter 8.) In some inflammatory conditions of the eye, this angle is obliterated, and there would be no place for the implant to lie. Prior to surgery, the doctor can learn whether the angle is open by examining the eye with a gonioscope.

If your anterior chamber angle is open, dilating your pupils is safe. Two kinds of eyedrops—Mydriacyl or Cyclogyl, and phenylephrine—are usually used. These drops work by temporarily paralyzing the muscles in the iris that make the pupil small and by stimulating the muscles that make the pupil big. The pupil enlarges to its greatest extent, facilitating a clear view of the back of the eye. Your doctor can then further examine the part of the cataract that is partly hidden by the iris, get an idea how much your pupil will dilate for your cataract surgery, and look at the retina, the fifth part of the eye examination. The drops will take about half an hour to work, so you'll need to return to the waiting room.

Retina Examination

An examination of the retina may be as important as the examination of the cataract. The results of both examinations will have a major effect on the decision to operate and the prognosis for improving sight. The retina, the membranelike lining of the back of the eye, is viewed through an ophthalmoscope. The usual ophthalmoscope is a hand-held instrument, something like a flashlight with lenses, through which the ophthalmologist focuses on the back of your eye. (Your medical doctor also uses the ophthalmoscope to uncover any effects of high blood pressure and diabetes in your eyes.) The problem with this instrument is that it does not emit a strong enough light to see through a cataract.

Another type of ophthalmoscope, the binocular indirect ophthalmoscope, is indispensable in evaluating a patient for cataract surgery. It emits an extremely strong light that, except with a very dense cataract, will allow an eye doctor a sufficiently clear view of the retina to predict whether it is normal. If the retina is not normal, removing the cataract may not improve vision enough to warrant an operation.

Several conditions, such as macular degeneration, fairly common in older patients and thought due to hardening of the arteries, weaken the retina and reduce vision. Vision loss from macular degeneration can sometimes be confused with that from cataracts, especially if the cataract is dense enough to prevent a clear view of the retina. The indirect ophthalmoscope is mounted on a headband, and with the lights out your eye doctor may look more like a coal miner than a physician. By having you look in different directions, he or she can examine the entire retina. The denser your cataract, the less clear will be the view of the retina, because the cataract will prevent him or her from looking in to the same extent it prevents you from looking out. By carefully studying your retina, your ophthalmologist will try to determine how much of your vision problem is due to retina trouble, if any, and how much due to the cataract.

The eye examination—including the history, refraction, external examination, slit-lamp examination, and retina examination—is now completed. If surgery is contemplated, several additional tests may be necessary at this time—the A-scan, keratometry, B-scan, endothelial cell count, glare, and Potential Acuity Meter tests.

A-scan

The A-scan measures the length of your eye by sound waves and is done to estimate the power or prescription of your implant. As we shall see in Chapter 8, almost all cataract surgery involves not only the removal of your cloudy lens, but its replacement with a clear, plastic lens—an implant or intraocular lens, which serves the same focusing function as does your own natural lens. Without an implant, your vision would be extremely blurred, requiring thick cataract glasses or a contact lens to restore sight.

The normal length of the eye—from the cornea, back through the pupil, through the lens (or cataract), through the vitreous, and through the retina—is about 24 millimeters, or approximately 1 inch. Since you cannot measure this with a ruler, the A-scan machine uses sound waves to measure the length of your eye—in scientific terms, its axial length. This measurement is used by your doctor to calculate the power of your implant; the shorter your eye, the stronger the implant has to be to bend the light rays to focus on your retina. "Short-eyed" people tend to be farsighted whereas "long-eyed" people are usually nearsighted. The length of your eye has no correlation with your height, only with your eyeglass prescription. In severe myopia, the strength of the implant, as calculated by the A-scan, may be so weak as to make an implant unnecessary.

Although the A-scan is quite accurate in measuring the length of your eye and determining the optimum power of your implant, no means is 100 percent accurate in determining whether you will need glasses for reading or distance after cataract surgery. Most patients will still need glasses for one or the other or even both after surgery, since small amounts of astigmatism, nearsightedness, or farsightedness often remain. The improvement in vision far outweighs the inconvenience of wearing glasses. The A-scan test does put you in a unique position, allowing you, with your doctor's advice, to choose between relying on distance glasses or reading glasses. The A-scan will give a reading of several prescriptions that can result from selecting a certain power of implant, and your ophthalmologist should discuss the choices before surgery. No patient should have an implant without a prior A-scan. (See Chapter 8 for more about this.)

Keratometry

Keratometry, a measurement of the curvature of the cornea, is also used to help calculate the power of the implant. The more curved your cornea, the more nearsighted will be your eye and the weaker the implant needs to be. The data from the A-scan and keratometer are fed into a small computer that calculates the strength of the implant needed to give you the best vision. We discuss this in greater detail in Chapter 8.

B-scan

The B-scan is an ultrasound test used in patients with a cataract too dense to permit any useful view of the retina with the binocular indirect ophthalmoscope. Operating successfully on a very dense cataract, only to discover that it hid a detached retina or severe macular degeneration, is frustrating for both patient and ophthalmologist. Even though the cataract operation was a success, the patient still will not see with that eye. The B-scan, more effectively than the A-scan, gives a picture of the eye behind the cataract. Although it cannot detect macular degeneration, it can alert the doctor to the presence of a retinal detachment. Your ophthalmologist will know if the B-scan ultrasound test is needed.

Endothelial Cell Count

The endothelial cell count is one of the best ways to determine the health of the cornea and to predict how it will stand up to cataract surgery. The endothelium is a single layer of cells lining the inside of the cornea, which is bathed in the aqueous fluid in the anterior chamber (the front part of the eye). These cells prevent the fluid inside your eye from entering the cornea, causing it to swell and lose clarity.

We are all born with a certain number of endothelial cells, and as we get older some of the cells die and are lost. The cornea has a very limited ability to make new cells and repair itself. A certain number of endothelial cells are needed to maintain a clear cornea and some of these cells—up to about 5 or 10 percent—are normally lost during cataract and implant surgery. If a person has only 50 percent of these endothelial cells left when cataract surgery is needed, and he or she loses another 15 or even 20 percent during the surgery, the person may have too few endothelial cells left to ensure a healthy cornea. The result may be a successful operation, but vision still hampered by a cloudy cornea. Such clouding can adversely and permanently affect eyesight, and a corneal transplant may be needed to replace the cloudy one. By using an instrument similar to the slit lamp, called an endothelial cell camera, your ophthalmologist can count, fairly accurately, the number of cells present in the endothelium. If the cell count is low—1,000 is about the lower limit of normal—your doctor can take special precautions during cataract surgery to minimize the risk of endothelial cell loss. With a very low cell count, such as 500, your doctor may anticipate that a corneal transplant will be needed in the future, and may recommend that a corneal transplant be combined with the cataract and implant operation. This "triple procedure"—cataract surgery, intraocular lens implant, and corneal transplant—will in effect save you a second operation later on.

Most people about to undergo cataract surgery do not need an endothelial cell count. Certain signs detected with the slit lamp will alert your doctor to perform the endothelial cell count, if necessary.

Glare Testing

A glare test attempts to gauge your true vision under battlefield conditions—in the real world of driving, walking, and working. Many patients with cataracts report disabling glare and blurred vision, especially outdoors, out of proportion to seemingly adequate vision as it is measured in a dark examining room. The effect of glare on your vision may best be measured by your eye doctor with a special glare tester. One such device, the Brightness Acuity Tester (BAT), was described on p. 18. Glare tests are somewhat controversial among ophthalmologists; some eye doctors feel it is merely a way of justifying doing more surgery, while others believe a glare test is a valuable means of getting a more accurate picture of the patient's symptoms in real life.

The Guyton-Minkowski Potential Acuity Meter

Will you see better after cataract surgery? This question is basic to all cataract surgery, because there is no need to have the operation unless it will improve your sight.

About 10 percent of patients with cataracts dense

enough to impair vision have macular degeneration that independently may be bad enough to impair their vision. Ophthalmologists and their patients thus are often faced with the question: Which is responsible for a patient's poor vision, the cataract or the retina? Just as the cataract prevents the patient from looking out, it may also prevent the doctor from looking in with enough clarity to eliminate retina trouble as the cause of impaired vision. The dilemma has been largely resolved by an ingeniously simple device called the Potential Acuity Meter (PAM), developed by two ophthalmologists at Johns Hopkins University, Dr. David L. Guyton and Dr. John S. Minkowski. The PAM, mounted on the slit lamp, projects an eye chart, via a tiny beam of light one-quarter the diameter of a pin, through minute clear areas of the cataract, directly onto the retina. You can then read the eye chart as if the cataract were not there. This indicates your potential for vision in the eye once the cataract is removed (and reassures you that your vision will indeed be a lot better after surgery). Although the PAM is not foolproof, it is a remarkable instrument.

__7__
Surgery

Until about twenty-five years ago, the topic of cataract surgery would have demanded only about one-third the space devoted to it in this chapter. There was essentially one type of operation, and implants were just coming out of the experimental stage. Most patients would end up with thick cataract glasses or a contact lens after spending two or three months recovering from surgery, with restrictions on bending, lifting, and many other daily activities.

Today the cataract operation has changed so much, and the events surrounding it have become so complex, that no matter how patiently and carefully your ophthalmologist explains cataract surgery, you may nonetheless find it difficult to make an intelligent decision about when to have surgery and what type of operation to have. You cannot leave the decision entirely in the hands of your eye doctor, as well meaning as he or she is, since cataract surgery is elective, rather than emergency surgery. Your evaluation of the doctor's advice, compared with the quality of your own symptoms, will greatly influence your decision on surgery. You will bear most of the responsibility for deciding when to have cataract surgery. This chapter will try to clear up the mystery surrounding cataract surgery and help you take some responsibility for your own well being by becoming a more informed patient. You must make a series of decisions based on the advice of your ophthalmologist and on your own feelings, whether they are gut feelings or feelings based on a careful, logical evaluation of your symptoms. The first is the decision to have surgery.

In the majority of cases, the decision to remove a cataract is based on your symptoms rather than on the appearance of the cataract during the slit-lamp examination. You, rather than the eye doctor, will know when that cataract is ready to come out. The newborn baby "knows" when the nine months are up and gives unmistakable warning signs that it is time to be delivered. The signs are not as definitive when a cataract is ready to be delivered, but they are discernible just the same if you understand what to look for.

You are ready for cataract surgery when you can no longer see well enough to do the things you enjoy, perform your daily activities in a satisfactory manner, and function adequately and happily. When you have cataracts and do not elect to have surgery, you have to accept the fact that although you can function adequately, you may not function optimally. You must make a trade-off, weighing your symptoms against the need for surgery. Often a person's decision to have surgery boils down to his or her philosophy. Knowing that a cataract operation is eventually unavoidable, some patients will "get it over with" and enjoy improved sight, while some will postpone it as long as possible.

If your diminished vision prevents you from functioning adequately, cataract surgery is necessary. Of course, what is adequate functioning for one person may be incapacitating misery for another. That is why the level of vision and the appearance of your cataract are less reliable signs of the need for surgery than your own state of happiness in the world. How well you drive a car, watch TV, or read a newspaper is more important than how well you read an eye chart. Only after balancing the history of poor vision against the appearance of the cataract and the level of eyesight can an ophthalmologist advise you either that it is time to have cataract surgery or that the symptoms are not bad enough to warrant an operation. In most cases, allowing a cataract to grow will not hurt your eye or make surgery more difficult later. You have plenty of time to reevaluate your life-style and decide how your reduced vision is altering it.

Ophthalmologists have accepted certain general guidelines to aid patients in determining when surgery is necessary. These guidelines pertain to the level of visual acuity in the affected eye. Certainly, surgery would never be done on an eye with a mild cataract that reduces vision only slightly to levels of 20/25 or 20/30. Vision of 20/40 is legal for driving in most states, so a cataract in each eye causing a drop from 20/20 to 20/40 would most likely be something you could put up with without much difficulty. Vision of 20/50 would be more difficult to live with, but many patients would not be too inconvenienced at this level. When vision is reduced to levels of 20/70 or 20/100 you cannot drive a car, cannot easily read a newspaper, and cannot look across the street without the sense of a haze or blur. At this level we generally start thinking seriously about cataract surgery. If both eyes are affected, most patients will go ahead and have surgery in the worse eye. Unless complications develop, cataract surgery is never performed on both eyes at the same time.

If vision is reduced to 20/200 or worse, which is legal blindness, your doctor will strongly recommend surgery. Patients I encounter with this level of vision from cataracts and who have not had surgery despite good advice are usually inordinately fearful of the operation or are denying their illness. It is frustrating to see a patient accept near blindness rather than have a thirty- or forty-five-minute operation, especially when there are thousands of blind patients for whom there is no treatment.

These general guidelines apply to the average patient with the average cataract, but many exceptions occur, from a small cataract that causes annoying, almost disabling, glare, to the blur from a small cataract that interferes with comfortable driving or reading. The more confident an eye surgeon feels about his or her own skills, the earlier he or she may, in good conscience, recommend you proceed with cataract surgery. If you are a sixty-year-old accountant or secretary, have a cataract in each eye, reducing your vision to 20/50, and cannot do your work, a cataract operation may be necessary even though your level of vision is not particularly incapacitating for household and leisure activities.

In rare instances a cataract may get so big and swollen that it blocks the free passage of fluid from the eye, causing a rise of intraocular pressure. This can lead to glaucoma, necessitating emergency cataract removal, not only to improve sight but to prevent blindness from glaucoma. A cataract can also grow to the point where any further growth will make removal more difficult, especially by the newer type of surgery, phacoemulsification. In this situation, surgery would be necessary for technical as well as visual reasons. Much more rarely, an extremely advanced cataract can rupture in the eye, causing considerable inflammation. As frightening as they sound, these situations are extremely uncommon, and usually occur only with a cataract so dense as to have already reduced vision to levels of hand motion or light perception.

You have decided to have cataract surgery. But which method of cataract surgery is best? Should you have the "old-fashioned" method, or the new one with space-age electronics, logic control, computerized function, and flashing lights? Do you want your cataract frozen, broken up, emulsified, or homogenized? Do you want a round implant or an oval one? Do you want one that folds in half or one that acts as a bifocal, possibly eliminating the need for glasses at all? This array of options may seem overwhelming, but after reading this book you will be fully able to understand them and the advice of your eye doctor.

There are three main types of cataract surgery: intracapsular, extracapsular, and phacoemulsification. In the intracapsular type, the entire cataract with its surrounding capsule is removed in one piece. In the extracapsular operation, the front of the capsule is opened, and the nucleus and cortex of the lens are removed separately, while the clear back part of the capsule is purposely left behind. Phacoemulsification (small-incision or no-stitch surgery) is a type of extracapsular cataract operation in which the cataract is liquefied (emulsified) and then sucked out, with the clear posterior capsule again left behind. We will examine all three methods to help determine which is best for you.

Before undergoing any type of cataract surgery, it is important that you have a thorough evaluation by your regular medical doctor. A physical examination, with chest X ray, cardiogram, and blood count, may detect problems such as high blood pressure and diabetes that can affect the surgery.

Intracapsular Cataract Extraction

In intracapsular cataract extraction, the standard form of cataract surgery from the early 1930s until the late 1970s, the entire cataractous lens—the hard nucleus in the center, the surrounding softer cortex, and the peachskinlike capsule enclosing it—are all removed in one piece. (See

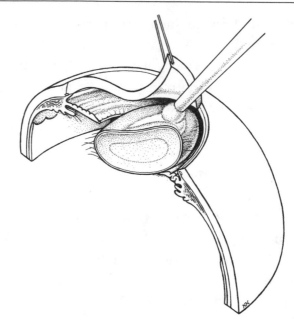

Figure 4   Intracapsular cataract extraction with iceball at tip of cryoprobe. The entire lens (capsule, cortex, nucleus) is removed in one piece.

Fig. 4.) The cataract is removed within its capsule, hence the name "intracapsular."

The intracapsular method, now popular only in undeveloped and third world countries, revolutionized cataract surgery because it allowed the cataract to be removed early, before it was totally white and opaque. This restored vision to thousands of people who would otherwise have had to wait and suffer until their cataracts were ripe enough to come out by the older, crude form of extracapsular surgery. The first generation of intraocular lenses in the late 1960s and early 1970s were designed to be used with intracapsular surgery. If you had cataract surgery in one eye and it was performed more than twenty years ago, it was most likely by the intracapsular method.

Intracapsular cataract extraction, with its higher complication rate over modern extracapsular cataract surgery, is rarely performed in the United States and in other countries with advanced forms of medical care.

Microsurgery, begun by eye surgeons in 1947, came into widespread use in ophthalmology in the early 1970s and made possible further advances in cataract surgery. Prior to the use of the operating microscope, eye surgery was done with the naked eye or with loupes-glasses with an attachment over each eye, which provided a small amount of magnification. Most ophthalmologists, myself included, first learned cataract surgery with loupes; only at the end of my residency did I learn the fundamentals of microsurgery. The operating microscope not only allows surgeons to see minute details only imagined before, but it allows surgeons to use finer instruments and sutures (stitches), heralding meticulous technique and a more successful operation. Although not critical in intracapsular surgery, an operating microscope is crucial to the success of the two current methods of cataract surgery—extracapsular and phacoemulsification.

Extracapsular Cataract Extraction

Extracapsular surgery began on April 8, 1745, when the great French ophthalmologist Jacques Daviel was performing his usual couching operation on a wigmaker called Farian. At that time couching was the only method known for removing cataracts and, indeed, the procedure dated back centuries before Christ. In couching, a needle is inserted through the white of the eye and into the lens from the side. The surgeon then uses the needle to push the cataract down out of the line of sight, allowing a clear pathway for light to enter the eye.

On this particular occasion, however, Daviel was unable to push the cataractous lens out of the center of the pupil and was about to face total failure. (The success rate for this operation was around 50 percent.) In what must have been a flash of inspiration and courage, if not near foolishness, he made an opening in the lower portion of the cornea, large enough to remove the cataract, then reached in with an instrument behind the cataract and brought the whole lens out of the eye. Although this had never been done before, the operation was a success and Farian, aided by thick cataract glasses, recovered to make many more wigs. By 1750 Daviel was convinced that his method was superior to couching, and in 1753 he delivered to the Royal Academy of Surgery a historic paper describing his results in 115 cataract operations. By 1756 he had performed 434 operations with only 50 failures, a much better record than in couching. What led up to the extraordinarily refined, beautifully orchestrated extracapsular cataract extraction of today was a long series of improvements in knowledge, instrumentation, and surgical technique. Today cataract surgery is one of the most successful operation performed on the human body. Let's see how a typical extracapsular extraction is done.

On the day of surgery, about one to one and a half hours before your operation, your pupil will be dilated to its widest extent by three or four applications of eyedrops, spaced about ten minutes apart. This series of drops is an important part of the whole operation and often makes the difference between a smooth operation and a difficult one. The more your cataract is exposed as the iris dilates, the easier the surgery will be. If your pupil is too small, your eye surgeon may have to enlarge it during surgery by excising a tiny portion of the iris, allowing better access to the cataract. This is especially true in patients with glaucoma, where antiglaucoma drops may cause the pupil to be permanently small. If you are going to have extracapsular surgery, your ophthalmologist will probably dilate your eye in the office and note beforehand the extent to which your pupil can be dilated. Special techniques can be used in patients with a small pupil, but a well-dilated pupil means easier surgery.

In extracapsular surgery, your cataract is removed in parts—first the front or anterior part of the capsule, followed by the hard central nucleus, and finally the soft cortex resting between the outer capsule and the inner nucleus. (See Fig. 5.) The back or posterior part of the capsule is intentionally left behind and helps support the implant in place. The relatively small incision, less than

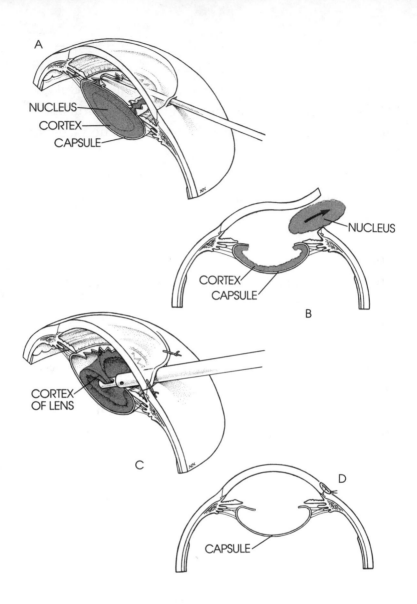

Figure 5   Extracapsular cataract extraction. *(a)* Beer-can openings are made into the front, or anterior, part of the capsule. *(b)* The nucleus is expressed out of the eye. *(c)* The cortex is sucked out. *(d)* The clear, posterior capsule remains.

half an inch, is big enough for the hard nucleus to be removed from the eye in one piece, while the remaining cortex is aspirated, or sucked out, through a small probe attached by tubes to a delicate irrigating/aspirating suction machine resembling a vacuum cleaner. A specially balanced sugar and mineral solution is irrigated into the eye at the same rate that the cortex is aspirated out of the eye, while delicate sensors in the probe maintain the normal shape and volume of the eye during cortex removal. This surgery requires both coordination and dexterity, since the surgeon will be using not only both hands to perform the surgery but both feet as well, one foot to work the foot pedal of the irrigating/aspirating "vacuum cleaner" and the other to work the foot pedal of the operating microscope, constantly adjusting focus and magnification. The surgeon will be doing all this while looking through the eyepieces of the microscope, relying on skillful eye-hand-foot coordination to orchestrate the surgery.

After learning extracapsular cataract surgery and performing the operation for a number of years, I had new respect for truck drivers and airplane pilots, whose hands and feet are constantly busy shifting gears, adjusting gauges, and working foot pedals while they adjust their focus and maintain a straight course. Although all this does sound complicated, extracapsular cataract extraction is a standard operation practiced by almost all eye surgeons, and has well over a 95 percent success rate.

Phacoemulsification:
Small-Incision or No-Stitch Cataract Surgery

The third method of cataract extraction, phacoemulsification (called phaco by many eye surgeons), was developed by Dr. Charles Kelman in 1967. In this variation of extracapsular surgery, the nucleus is not removed in one piece but is broken up and liquified (emulsified) by ultrasound. A similar type of irrigating/aspirating machine used for extracapsular surgery is used for phacoemulsification, with the addition of a handheld probe tipped with a hollow titanium tip. The doctor activates a foot pedal that causes the tip to vibrate back and forth 40,000 times per second, emulsifying or breaking up the hard nucleus like a jackhammer breaking up concrete. As the cataract is being emulsified, fluid travels from an IV bottle into the eye through tubing surrounding the hollow titanium tip. The fluid mixes with the emulsified remnants of the cataract and leaves through separate tubing. Sensors in the probe maintain a constant balance between fluid entering the eye and fluid aspirating out of the eye.

What makes phaco even more attractive than previous methods is that, rather than an incision big enough to remove the half-inch nucleus in one piece, in phacoemulsification the entire incision needs only to be big enough to accommodate the ultrasonic probe, about one-eighth of an inch. The healing process is consequently quicker, and less astigmatism usually results.

A lot of publicity, generally unfavorable, attended the early use of Kelman's procedure, because initially the complication rate was higher than with other methods. As more and more ophthalmologists gained experience with phacoemulsification, the results steadily improved, although until recently many eye surgeons were still reluctant to attempt it. In the mid-1980s, improvements in technique completely changed the way phacocmulsification was performed, making it so safe and successful that by 1995 close to 80 percent of ophthalmologists will prefer phacoemulsification as their method of cataract surgery, while 20 percent still prefer standard extracapsular cataract extraction. Those eye surgeons who perform phacoemulsification appreciate the ability to remove an entire cataract through a tiny incision.

Since your surgeon's preference will have a direct bearing on your cataract operation, you should understand which type of operation may be best for you and know which is preferred by your eye surgeon. If your ophthalmologist does only extracapsular cataract surgery and not phacoemulsification, you needn't feel you ought to change doctors, since results from the two procedures are about equal in the long run. Phacoemulsification does have some advantages, as we shall see, but well-qualified eye doctors disagree about whether these advantages are worthwhile.

The recent rise in popularity of phacoemulsification is a result of improved safety and a high degree of patient satisfaction. The main problems with the older method of phacoemulsification were inflammation and clouding of the cornea from the probe's ultrasonic vibration and energy as it liquefied the nucleus, in close proximity to the

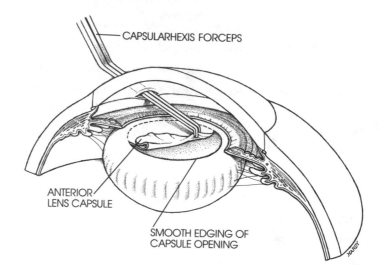

CAPSULARHEXIS FORCEPS

ANTERIOR LENS CAPSULE

SMOOTH EDGING OF CAPSULE OPENING

Figure 6   The smooth, round capsularhexis is better suited for phacoemulsification than the jagged cut of the capsulotomy.

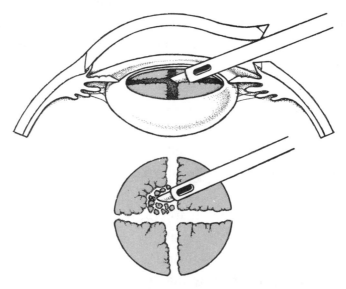

Figure 7   In the popular phacoemulsification method known as divide-and-conquer, the nucleus is sculpted into four pieces and each piece is then emulsified.

inside surface of the cornea. Safety improved in the early 1980s, with the development of Healon and other visco-elastic substances. These compounds, initially made from rooster cockscombs and used in horse racing to cushion horses' knee joints, were adapted for use in eye surgery to cushion the cornea and protect it from damage.

It wasn't until the late 1980s that several ophthalmologists, including the inventive Dr. Howard Gimbel of Calgary, Canada, devised methods to emulsify the nucleus more safely. Gimbel first devised an improved method of opening the front capsule, making phaco much safer. This technique, called capsulorhexis, is recognized as one of the most important contributions to cataract surgery in the last decade. Rather than opening the anterior capsule in the standard saw-toothed fashion, which involved making ten or twenty jagged openings in a circle around the capsule (see Fig. 5a), Dr. Gimbel used a controlled tearing method to make a smooth circular opening, leaving no irregular edges (see Fig. 6). This smooth opening, about ¼ inch in diameter, made the capsule much stronger, and more resistant to tearing during phacoemul-sification. (See Fig. 6.) Using the phaco probe like a sculptor with a chisel, Gimbel further improved the safety of phacoemulsification by first dividing the nucleus into four smaller, more manageable pieces and then safely emulsifying each small piece. (See Fig. 7.) In performing cataract surgery in this divide-and-conquer fashion, Gimbel was able to work farther away from the cornea and use less potentially damaging ultrasonic energy, minimizing any chance of cornea damage.

Other ophthalmologists, such as Dr. Paul Koch of War-wick, Rhode Island, devised their own methods of sculpting the nucleus into smaller and smaller pieces. The object of these new and revised forms of phacoemulsification was to safely sculpt the nucleus into smaller pieces before the main emulsification was completed. This technique required less ultrasonic energy to emulsify the nucleus making the operation much safer. Divide and Conquer, Chip and Flip, Spin and Thin, and Spring Surgery are all names to describe the various new techniques used in phacoemulsification. They all have in common the sequential removal of the cataract through a tiny incision, about ⅛ inch or the width of a match head.

The faster healing resulting from the small incision benefits the patient in several ways. The redness and inflammation normally present after cataract surgery disappear in two or three weeks rather than the six to eight weeks of extracapsular cataract surgery, and the patient is able to stop using eyedrops and get new glasses a lot sooner. But shortened healing time is not the only advantage of phacoemulsification. What really put phacoemulsification on the map were two other developments: no-stitch surgery and small-incision implants. We will discuss the former in this chapter; small-incision implants are discussed fully in the next chapter.

Many patients do not know or appreciate that removing the cataract and inserting an implant is only half the battle for the eye doctor. His or her job is not just to remove the cataract but to restore your sight. The occurrence of astigmatism after surgery may limit your visual recovery from an otherwise perfect cataract operation. Astigmatism, or an irregular cornea, occurs because the stitches used in cataract surgery pull on the cornea slightly, causing the round cornea to become slightly oval. This change in shape, from that of a basketball to that of a football, results in astigmatism, usually accompanied by a similar amount of farsightedness or nearsightedness.

Although some astigmatism is sometimes unavoidable, due to the vagaries of healing of the eye, high degrees of astigmatism are not desirable and are more difficult to correct with glasses than milder degrees of astigmatism. In general, the smaller the incision or opening to remove a cataract, the fewer sutures are needed to close the incision and the less astigmatism is produced. When phacoemulsification became popular in the mid-1980s, its smaller incision produced less astigmatism than extracapsular cataract extraction, but it still resulted in some.

Starting in the late 1980s, ophthalmologists, obsessed with eliminating any induced astigmatism from cataract surgery, made a series of innovative changes in the location of the incision and the number of sutures used to close it. Several eye surgeons, including Dr. Stuart Cole of Long Beach, California, moved the incision away from the more delicate cornea onto the sclera, where sutures exert much less pulling and give less astigmatism. Dr. John Shepherd of Las Vegas, Nevada, soon found that only one stitch, rather than the customary three or four, was all that was necessary to seal the incision in the sclera, hence the popular term for this variation of phacoemulsification, "one-stitch surgery."

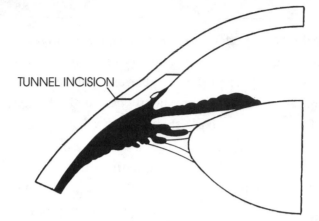

TUNNEL INCISION

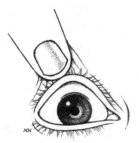

10MM LIMBAL INCISION
FOR EXTRASCAPSULAR SURGERY

5MM TUNNEL INCISION
FOR PHACOEMULSIFICATION

Figure 8   Scleral tunnel.

Dr. Michael McFarland of Pine Bluff, Arkansas, took this innovation one step further and is credited with starting "no-stitch" cataract surgery in which all sutures and, in effect, all astigmatism are eliminated. In this variation of phacoemulsification, McFarland started the incision in the usual location in the sclera, and then tunneled under it into the cornea, ending the incision in a self-sealing corneal flap. (See Fig. 8.) The architecture of this incision made the wound watertight without the need for sutures. Although astigmatism after phacoemulsification is almost the same whether the surgeon uses no stitches or one or even several, the no-stitch technique with a scleral tunnel, self-sealing incision is a major advance in rapidly restoring sight to patients with a cataract. McFarland received the 1992 Innovators Award from the Irish-American Ophthalmological Society for his development of sutureless cataract surgery.

Many eye surgeons quickly adopted the no-stitch technique, while others, performing the identical operation, felt safer adding one or several stitches, fearing complications such as infection. Many other ophthalmologists feel strongly that standard extracapsular surgery gives results equally as good as does phacoemulsification, although recovery takes somewhat longer and unwanted astigmatism must be controlled or eliminated by removing selected stitches about six weeks after surgery. Six months or a year after surgery, there is generally little difference in the results from extracapsular cataract surgery and phacoemulsification. Even if your ophthalmologist prefers phacoemulsification, not all patients are good candidates for this operation. A very hard, advanced cataract may be difficult to emulsify, making extracapsular surgery a better choice. A poorly dilated pupil may make phacoemulsification difficult. Your ophthalmologist can tell you if you are a good candidate for phacoemulsification.

Besides the tunnel incision, with its quicker healing and decreased astigmatism, another boost in popularity for phaco came from the introduction of small-incision implants, a technological breakthrough in implant design. These implants were developed to complement and retain the advantages of the small incision of phacoemulsification, so that the 3-millimeter (1/10th inch) tiny phaco incision would not have to be enlarged to 7 millimeters (1/4 inch) to accommodate a standard-size implant. Implants were developed that could fold in half and fit through a 3 or 4-millimeter opening; oval implants, measuring 5 by 6 millimeters, fit through a 5-millimeter opening. Ophthalmologists are obsessed with millimeters, and will go to any length to save a few millimeters—and healing time— for their patients. This is high-tech surgery in spades! More about implants in Chapter 8.

Anesthesia

Since anesthesia is what makes the operation possible, it is important to understand the different types available. The type of anesthetic you will have depends mainly on your preference and that of your surgeon. Although being

completely asleep under general anesthesia sounds inviting, most ophthalmologists prefer local anesthesia, justi-
fiably believing that it is safer to numb only your eye than
your whole body.

LOCAL ANESTHESIA

The object of local anesthesia during an eye operation
is not only to numb the eye and block pain, but to prevent
you from closing and moving your eye during surgery.
Your eye surgeon or an anesthesiologist will administer
the anesthetic. Even if your ophthalmologist gives you the
local anesthetic, as occurs in most cataract operations, an
anesthesiologist will usually be at your side to check your
blood pressure, pulse, breathing, and cardiogram during
the operation. He or she will start an intravenous (IV) drip
with a mixture of salt water and sugar, not so much to
feed you, but to be ready should the need arise to give
you medication through the IV tubing. Should you become extra anxious or develop blood pressure or heart
problems, the anesthesiologist can administer medication
through the IV without disturbing you or your surgeon.
Having an anesthesiologist take care of you will not only
benefit your general health, but it will also allow your
surgeon to concentrate fully on the surgery at hand. Good
anesthesia with a relaxed patient adds significantly to the
successful outcome of the surgery.

After you have received a mild sedative, usually through
the IV tubing, two injections are generally given—one
near your ear to numb the facial nerve and to prevent
your eyelids from closing, and a retrobulbar block near

your eye to completely numb your eye and to prevent all movement of the eye muscles. There is absolutely no injection into the eye, as many patients fear. Although the injections may sound like instruments of torture, they are safe and only mildly uncomfortable. Occasionally the retrobulbar injection leaves a black-and-blue mark around the eyelid; in rare cases, the needle may injure a small blood vessel behind the eye, causing localized bleeding. We will discuss more about the administration of the anesthetic in Chapter 10.

In order to test the effectiveness of the anesthetic injection, your eye surgeon will ask you to look up, down, left, and right, and to close your eyes tightly. When no movement of your eye or lids is seen and you have failed all these commands, you are ready for surgery. You will feel absolutely no pain.

Once the actual surgery starts, it is not as critical as you might think that you be absolutely still and not talk; but it is certainly helpful to interrupt your own eye surgery as little as possible. The sedative will usually make you relaxed, calm, and even sleepy. It should not induce a deep sleep; upon awakening from deep sleep patients are somewhat disoriented and may move excessively. Your ophthalmologist will probably prefer that you be undersedated or not sedated at all rather than oversedated. After the operation, you will have a brief rest period in a recovery area, change back into your clothes, and return home. You will experience some discomfort when the anesthetic wears off, usually starting two to three hours after surgery. With a good local anesthetic and well-performed surgery, the total effect on your system is almost like a visit to the dentist, a not-unpleasant comparison I hope.

GENERAL ANESTHESIA

General anesthesia means you are unconscious and completely asleep. An anesthesiologist will start an intravenous drip through which he will add a sedative, such as Pentothal, to induce sleep. He will then pass an endotracheal tube into your windpipe, through which you will breathe a mixture of anesthetic gases causing you to remain completely asleep and pain free. After you awaken you will go to the recovery room for several hours, where a nurse will check your vital signs (blood pressure, pulse, and respiration) until most of the anesthetic has worn off. During this time you may be mildly nauseated from the anesthetic and may have a slight sore throat from the endotracheal tube. This quickly passes, and by that evening or the next morning you will be back to normal. Although general anesthesia can be given in outpatient surgery, it is more common to have patients stay in the hospital overnight while the anesthetic wears off completely.

You will not need any injection to anesthetize your eye locally and will not even be slightly awake or aware of surgery. The disadvantage of general anesthesia is that your whole body is affected by the anesthetic. Elderly patients, who often have other health problems, such as hypertension and heart disease, should avoid general anesthesia if possible. Although general anesthesia is usually completely safe, there is a general mortality rate of 1 in

10,000. This number is somewhat higher in elderly, frail patients. I reserve a general anesthetic for those few patients who are excessively anxious and want to feel nothing and know nothing. It is wise to discuss anesthesia with your eye surgeon when you decide to have surgery.

Surgical Setting

Where should you have your operation? Fifteen or twenty years ago, this question would have sounded somewhat ridiculous, as the only place to have cataract surgery was at a hospital, with a required stay of several days. You would be admitted on day one, have surgery on day two, and go home on anywhere from day three to day seven. Since the first edition of this book, inpatient cataract surgery has become the exception, requiring prior approval from Medicare and similar health-insurance plans and, in effect, "a note from your doctor" explaining why you are too ill to have surgery in the now standard ambulatory setting. In the current climate in which American health care is dictated more by budgets and political considerations and less by compassion and decency, elderly frail patients with everything from heart disease to severe diabetes to many other maladies are being required to have cataract surgery as outpatients or pay for the surgery privately. Insurance companies discourage or deny coverage for even a one-night hospital stay. If your ophthalmologist recommends inpatient surgery, he or she will invariably receive a call from your health-insurance representative asking to justify this decision. Final approval will depend on the medical indications each patient has for inpatient surgery.

In fairness to our health-care system, which is probably the best in the world, outpatient surgery—no matter how old the patient—is usually preferable to an overnight stay in a hospital filled with sick patients. However, many patients who live alone feel uneasy spending the night after surgery at home by themselves. Although the thought of returning home after surgery may seem objectionable or radical, you probably do not need medical care the first night, and will generally feel more comfortable in your own home.

In the past ten to fifteen years, most hospitals have greatly expanded their facilities for ambulatory surgery, including cataract surgery, in response to rising costs and changes in health-care reimbursement. A federally funded study in 1978 found that as much as a 50 percent savings was possible with ambulatory surgery, prompting new interest. By 1990, according to an American Hospital Association analysis, almost every hospital in the country was equipped for outpatient surgery, and for the first time ever, over half the operations in the country were ambulatory. Today, well over 95 percent of cataract patients will have their surgery on an outpatient basis, and be home in time for dinner and the six o'clock news.

If your cataract operation is to be performed on an outpatient basis, you will most likely report to the hospital's ambulatory surgical area on the morning of the surgery and will be escorted to the operating room. Almost all ambulatory cataract surgery is performed with a local anesthetic. After surgery and a brief rest you will change back into your clothes and return home, using your unoperated eye to see. You may be slightly unsteady from the sedative, so you should not drive or walk by yourself right after surgery. It is wise to have a friend or relative accompany you home. Although ambulatory surgery is ideal for most patients, it is not for everybody. If you are anxious and prefer the security and comfort of the inpatient hospital setting, speak to your doctor.

Freestanding ambulatory surgical centers, sometimes called surgicenters, are smaller in scale than hospitals. About 20 percent of all outpatient surgery is performed in a surgicenter. One of the first of these centers was established in Phoenix, Arizona, in 1969 by Dr. Wallace Reed and Dr. John Ford. There are now about 1,500 surgicenters throughout the country. Designed only for outpatient surgery, they are usually ultramodern, with wall-to-wall carpeting, piped-in music, comfortable lounge areas, and a friendly, efficient, and courteous staff. Most of the surgery performed at these centers lasts less than two to three hours, and recovery takes less than four hours. This general policy is to ensure that only suitable types of surgery are done at these centers. Medicare, Blue Cross, and most other health insurance plans will cover same-day ambulatory surgery performed in surgicenters. Most surgicenters must be licensed by a state or national accrediting body, but licensing and regulation are inconsistent and differs from state to state. Most states require annual inspection of ambulatory surgical facilities and require that a surgicenter be within a certain distance from a hospital, should an emergency arise. Oregon state representative Ron Wyden, head of a House subcommittee that has studied the safety of nonhospital clinics and surgicenters for the past four years, says as reported in the *New York Times*, July 1, 1992, that the quality of care in these centers is generally good. However, he will soon introduce legislation to require stricter licensing and more regulation.

Surgery in an operating room in your doctor's office, a newer, more recent setting for ambulatory cataract surgery, is another option also approved by Medicare and other health insurance providers. This "one-stop shopping" does have its advantages: Having your surgery in a familiar setting with familiar staff may make you feel more relaxed and comfortable. The disadvantage is that having the surgery in the same office where you get your glasses checked may make you equate the two procedures. Although your operation is performed in the office, it is the same operation whether you stay in the hospital for one or two nights or have it in the hospital on an ambulatory basis or in a surgicenter. An operating room in a doctor's office must adhere to the same standards and regulation as one in a hospital or surgicenter. Most patients have no strong preference for where their surgery is performed as long as it is well done and as pain free as possible.

8

Seeing Again: Glasses, Contact Lenses, and Implants

The operation is over, a patch and plastic shield are taped over your eye, and you are relaxing at home on your sofa or having coffee in your kitchen. An hour or two ago the sight out of your eye was veiled by a cataractous haze, which is now gone forever. Now that the lens in your eye is gone, and light has a clear pathway into it, what will focus the light into a clear image? The lens accounted for about one-third of the refractive power of the eye, and without it you will fall that much short of receiving a clear image.

An eye without a lens cannot focus and is said to be *aphakic*, from the Greek *a* for "without" and *phakos* for "lentil seed" or anything similarly shaped, such as the human lens. Your cataract operation transformed your eye from phakic (with a lens) to aphakic (without a lens). If cataracts have been removed from both eyes, you are known to ophthalmologists as a bilateral aphake. Cataract surgery in only one eye makes you a monocular aphake.

The correction of aphakia—how the eye sees again after cataract surgery—is achieved in three ways: glasses, contact lenses, or intraocular lenses. You should understand the differences between the three methods to fully appreciate the miraculous advance in sight restoration provided by intraocular lenses, the method preferred by ophthalmologists throughout the world. In some ways the method you and your doctor select to correct your impending aphakia is more important than the method you selected to remove the cataract. Once the operation is over, you will never have to worry about a cataract in that eye again, since cataracts can never grow back. But the way you see with that eye will be with you as long as you live, so the subject of implants is an important one. This chapter will help you understand the three choices, and why, with rare exceptions, eyeglasses are the worst choice and implants the best. Contact lens correction after cataract surgery falls somewhere in between, and is usually used only in special circumstances.

Glasses

Glasses were the only means of correcting aphakia up to about forty years ago, when contact lenses became available. If your parents or grandparents wore glasses that looked about an inch thick and made their eyes look twice their size, chances are they had had cataract surgery and were wearing aphakic glasses. People did not complain much about glasses then, because at that time they had to wait to have surgery until, almost blind, both cataracts were ripe enough and one could be removed. Any vision was better than that, and patients were generally satisfied with glasses. However, as surgery became more sophisticated and cataracts began to be removed with the intracapsular technique before becoming totally ripe, patients became more and more unhappy with aphakic glasses. All thick cataract glasses have several problems, which sometimes outweigh the vision problems of the original cataract.

MAGNIFICATION

Cataract glasses magnify objects about 25 percent, causing them to appear bigger and nearer. The newly aphakic patient may pour cream onto the table rather than into the coffee cup, seeing the cup about two inches closer than it really is. The whole environment is also magnified, which can cause you to feel disoriented. Surgery in only one eye may result in an especially disturbing problem because the thick cataract glass over the operated eye has to be balanced by an equally thick cataract glass over the nonoperated eye. This allows good vision in the operated eye but intentionally blurs out the vision in the nonoperated eye. If the nonoperated eye is not blocked out and has a regular eyeglass instead, the brain will get a 25 percent bigger image from the operated eye than from the nonoperated eye, resulting in jarring, intractable double vision. Because this is as intolerable as the original cataract, it is inadvisable to combine a cataract glass over the operated eye with a regular glass over the nonoperated other eye. That is why when glasses were the only available correction for aphakia, a cataract in only one eye, however advanced, would generally not be removed until the second eye had a moderately advanced cataract as well so that after the first, ripe cataract was removed, the second eye wouldn't be affected much by being blocked out by a balancing eyeglass lens.

Also, thirty or forty years ago it was common for a patient to enter the hospital and have both cataracts removed a few days apart. Both cataracts progressed to a fairly ripe degree of maturity, both were removed, and the patient saw with both eyes again. But if a patient needed a mature cataract removed from one eye while the other eye was normal, he would not want to have his normal 20/20 eye blocked out by a cataract glass, no matter how well he saw out of his operated eye. In this case he would continue using his good eye and let the operated eye go uncorrected by glasses. Vision would feel much more natural from the unoperated eye, even if both eyes saw 20/20. The operated eye would be a sort of spare, ready to be called into service if and when the normal eye developed a cataract.

DISTORTION

If your grandparents or parents were finally able to adapt to the magnification problem of cataract glasses, they would still have had to contend with distortion, another annoying feature of aphakic spectacles. The thickness and curve of the cataract glass results not only in magnification of objects but in unequal magnification, which causes distortion. This distortion is most distressing when looking in any direction other than straight ahead; the farther you look to the right or left through a cataract glass, the more distortion and blurring you get. Aphakic patients corrected by glasses must quickly learn to turn their head rather than their eyes when looking to either side.

LIMITED VISUAL FIELD

A marked narrowing of the visual field is still another annoying change in vision caused by thick cataract glasses. Through cataract glasses only a small tunnel of vision is clear in front of you, similar to vision through binoculars. Worse yet, the strong cataract glass bends light rays so much that some rays from objects don't even enter the eye and are bent past it. The resulting circular blind area, called a *ring scotoma*, in the visual field of patients with cataract glasses corresponds to the circular edge of the cataract glass. Wherever patients look, the roving ring scotoma follows them like a shadow, blocking out part of their peripheral vision.

JACK-IN-THE-BOX PHENOMENON

Another problem plaguing cataract glass wearers is the Jack-in-the-box phenomenon—the annoying tendency of objects, hidden by the ring scotoma, to pop suddenly in and out of view as the wearers move their eyes away from the center of the glasses.

In the days when glasses were the only means to correct aphakic vision, Dr. Arthur Linksz, a renowned Hungarian ophthalmologist, wisely said, "the first complication of cataract surgery is aphakia." Fortunately most patients adapted to the vagaries of cataract glasses quite well and welcomed the improved sight despite the limitations of the glasses. Dr. Robert Welsh, inventor of the Welsh four-drop cataract glass, contributed to their satisfaction when he created a thinner, lighter, and better-looking aphakic lens, giving less magnification and distortion and a wider visual field.

Contact Lenses

Before intraocular lenses became available, contact lenses —hard, gas permeable, and soft—improved the quality of life for thousands of aphakic patients.

In the 1950s and 1960s, hard contact lenses so revolutionized the correction of vision after cataract surgery that thousands of people put down their thick glasses and learned how to place those hard, tiny plastic disks on their corneas. Gone was the 25 percent magnification, the distortion, the scotoma, the Jack-in-the-box phenomenon. Vision was back to normal, or almost so, and patients were a lot happier. Contact lenses, unlike glasses, gave much more natural vision, enabling patients thwarted by a cataract in only one eye to have that cataract removed without waiting for another to develop in the second eye. The brain is able to adjust much more easily to the 7 percent magnification of the contact lens, so that the non-operated eye no longer needed to be blocked out as it did with cataract glasses. Patients hampered by a cataract in only one eye, coping with the lack of depth perception and difficulty in coordination caused by the cataract, could regain normal vision after surgery by using a contact lens. In spite of these obvious advantages, however, contact lenses have several disadvantages.

SENSITIVITY

Although well motivated, some patients cannot adjust to a contact lens and never overcome the initial irritation. The cornea loses some of its sensitivity following cataract extraction; but in spite of this, many patients have difficulty adjusting to the presence of hard contact lenses. Gas-permeable lenses, developed in the early 1980s, look and feel like regular hard contact lenses but are made of a plastic that allows more oxygen to get to the cornea. These are more comfortable than hard contact lenses, and have made it possible for many more aphakic patients to wear a contact lens. If you have tried a hard contact lens in the past but couldn't get used to it, perhaps one of the newer gas-permeable materials will help you.

Soft contact lenses, introduced by Bausch & Lomb in 1971, were supposed to be much more comfortable and allow more patients to correct their aphakia without resorting to glasses. While the soft lens material, hard and brittle when dry, but swollen soft like a sponge when wet, is generally much more comfortable and can be worn for a longer period of time, it has several drawbacks.

LENS CARE

Maintenance and care of soft lenses are somewhat more involved than with hard lenses. Because they are porous, the soft lenses absorb the normal mucus, dirt, and protein in your tears and need to be not only cleaned every day as do hard lenses, but sterilized as well. This used to require heating the lenses in a special heater, but is now done with prepared solutions.

VISION

Vision is often unacceptably poor when corrected by a soft contact lens, usually because of uncorrected astigmatism. The astigmatism present after cataract surgery is due to an irregularity in the cornea from one suture being tighter than another or one part of the cornea healing differently from another part. A hard contact lens acts like a new, perfectly smooth cornea, while a soft contact lens more or less molds to the cornea, repeating most of the imperfections present. It is not unusual for patients to wear a soft contact lens to avoid thick cataract glasses, over which they will wear regular glasses to correct their astigmatism. Improved lens design has resulted in better-fitting, more comfortable soft contact lenses, as well as some that can specifically correct mild to moderate degrees of astigmatism. Soft lenses can now be custom made in almost any prescription.

HANDLING

Many patients have a great deal of difficulty handling a contact lens. Patients with arthritis or Parkinson's disease may lack the coordination and dexterity necessary to manipulate contact lenses, making it almost impossible for them to use a contact lens on a regular basis.

Switching from a hard to a soft contact lens does not solve the handling problem, and in many ways a soft lens is more difficult to insert and remove than a hard or gas-permeable lens.

A major breakthrough in the treatment of aphakia was the introduction in the late 1970s of the extended-wear soft contact lens (EWSCL). This lens, when wet, becomes up to 79 percent water; in contrast, a daily wear soft contact lens becomes about 40 percent water. The high water content and thinness of the EWSCL allows enough oxygen to travel to the cornea so that even during sleep, with the eyes closed, the eye gets enough oxygen. Continuous wear is possible for months at a time, although lens removal once a week is advisable.

It was with some trepidation that I fit my first patient with an extended-wear soft contact lens. I remember awakening in the middle of the night half expecting a phone call to report a bad result. The next morning I was greeted by a happy patient who also awoke during the night. For the first time since having both cataracts removed, he had the same good vision in the middle of the night as in the middle of the day.

But several problems still remain for extended soft lens wearers:

LENS LOSS

One of the most frustrating problems is loss of the lens. If you have ever gone to bed with your lenses in, only to awaken with one or both of them on your pillow or cheek, you know how annoying and perplexing this can be. Your eye doctor may try several different lenses—testing tighter or looser fits from several different companies—only to have the lenses drop out again. The exact cause of this is not known, although it is probably related to how well your eyelids close during sleep and to the moistness of your cornea, rather than to the fit of the lens.

DEPOSITS

One of the worst problems is the surface buildup of material that coats and clouds the lens, causing blurred vision and irritation. We all have protein, mucus, and minerals in our tears and on our eye, and these substances can accumulate on the lens and cloud it, in much the same way changes from age in the human lens cloud it and cause a cataract. Some patients may be able to wear a lens for even a year without any clouding, while others will cloud up a lens in several weeks or even days. The usual cleaning agents for soft lenses are often ineffective in removing these deposits, and replacing the lens with a new one is the only answer. Annoying deposits can come from blepharitis, a common, often unrecognized inflammation of the oil glands in the edge of the lid. If you have this problem and have not been successful in wearing a soft contact lens, ask your eye doctor about treatment for the lid problem. More successful contact lens wear should follow.

INFECTION

Although the safety of extended-wear soft lenses has been proven through clinical trials of thousands of patients, on very rare occasions serious eye infections can develop. Many patients who wear contact lenses will develop conjunctivitis (pinkeye), a mild, superficial infection of the conjunctiva, the membrane covering the white of the eye. This clears quite readily by discontinuing lens wear and using antibiotic eyedrops. A much less common but much more serious infection can occur on the cornea. This infection, called a corneal ulcer, is uncommon but potentially serious. Symptoms of pain, redness, and discharge associated with contact lens wear may mean a corneal ulcer. If the lens is removed and prompt eye care sought, permanent scarring of the cornea and loss of vision can usually be avoided.

Implants

Although contact lenses helped thousands of patients regain clear, natural vision after cataract surgery, many more patients could not adapt to a hard lens, could not handle a daily wear soft lens, and were not successful with an extended-wear lens. While many ophthalmologists retained their initial enthusiasm for contact lenses, others took a radically different course in pursuit of the intraocular lens (IOL). This quarter-inch plastic lens, inserted into the eye during cataract surgery, stirred more controversy than any other subject in ophthalmology and perhaps in all of medicine. The pioneers of intraocular lenses were reproached by their colleagues as radicals, maligned by consumer groups for risking patients' welfare in unproven surgery, and regulated by the federal government, which was unconvinced of the benefits of implants. Unshaken, they persevered in their belief that the best correction for an eye about to lose a cataractous lens was the insertion of a clear intraocular lens. Revolutionary ideas tend to be accepted slowly, and the idea that an intraocular lens could be safely used to correct aphakia was no exception. Today there is no doubt of the superiority of the intraocular lens in achieving the quality of vision present in an eye before the cataract developed.

The idea of replacing the human lens with an artificial one dates back to 1776, when Casanova, whose amorous adventures are legend, described a meeting with the Italian oculist Tadini, who showed him tiny crystal lenses that could replace the human lens. Casaamata, an Italian ophthalmologist who lived in Dresden around 1795, was the first to actually try this. Unfortunately, the glass lens immediately sank to the bottom of the eye and the patient had to wear spectacles from then on.

The modern age of intraocular lens implantation began on November 29, 1949, at the Thomas Hospital in London, where Dr. Harold Ridley implanted an artificial lens into the eye of a forty-five-year-old woman. His idea was inspired by a medical student, who, while watching Ridley complete a successful cataract extraction, innocently asked whether the doctor had forgotten to insert a new clear lens. The student had never seen a cataract operation before and thought it only common sense to replace the cataract with a clear lens. It is a tribute to Dr. Ridley that he did not dismiss the idea as nonsense but began to think about the feasibility of an artificial lens inside the eye. Further study led Ridley to select a plastic, polymethyl-methacrylate (PMMA) as the material from which to make the implant. The plastic canopies of British Spitfire air-planes were made of PMMA, and during the early part of the Battle of Britain in World War II, enemy gunfire downed many British planes. Fragments of the shattered canopy occasionally lodged in the eyes of pilots, and in those cases where it was more prudent to leave the plastic in the eye than risk removing it, the plastic appeared to be well tolerated and did no harm. Since the eyes of these injured pilots were able to tolerate PMMA, Ridley cor-rectly reasoned that it would be an ideal substance for an intraocular lens. His historic operation was a technical success, but owing to an error in the calculation of the strength of the implant, which was custom-made for the patient's prescription, the patient was left extremely near-sighted. Her eyesight was corrected to 20/60 later on with thick glasses. Ridley attempted a second implant, on Au-gust 23, 1950, and the operation led to a similar result. Although there were a few successes, Ridley abandoned his procedure in 1960 because of a high rate of complica-tions. The implant, placed behind the iris into the posterior chamber of the eye, often dislocated and fell to the bottom of the eye where it often had to be removed, or led to severe inflammation and glaucoma.

From 1950 to 1960 most of the great eye surgeons of

Europe tried to improve upon Ridley's results but had limited success. During this discouraging implant-of-the-month period there were dozens of different designs, each named after the ophthalmologist who designed it, each trying to solve the problems of past designs. Each one failed, either by moving out of place or causing excessive inflammation. Implant surgery and those who performed it became synonymous with recklessness, irresponsibility, and disaster. The noted Colombian ophthalmologist José Barraquer, one of the most respected eye surgeons of his time, implanted 493 lenses from 1954 to 1960, and eventually had to remove 250 of them because of complications.

Credit for saving the idea of implant surgery from oblivion goes to three men—Peter Choyce of England, Edward Epstein of South Africa, and the recognized father of early implant surgery, Cornelius Binkhorst of the Netherlands. These three men, working independently, were convinced of the potential benefit of implants, and were imaginative and innovative enough to design improved implants that worked. The Choyce lens, the Epstein lens, and the Binkhorst lens were used throughout Europe from around 1955 to 1965, when they were cautiously accepted by a few "radical" eye surgeons in the United States. Over the next fifteen years, as results and implant design steadily improved in the United States, implant surgery grew in popularity until, by 1980, over 75 percent of all cataract operations involved intraocular lens implantation. In 1993 the number approaches 100 percent.

FDA STUDY

The success of implants is due to the opthalmologists, who believed in the idea, and to their patients, who understood the risks and benefits of implants and chose to go ahead—frequently against the advice of more conservative ophthalmologists and many consumer groups, including Ralph Nader and his Citizen's Watch Group in the late 1960s and early 1970s. It wasn't until a U.S. Food and Drug Administration (FDA) study found implants to be safe and effective that they gained wide acceptance. In May 1976, during the height of interest in the field of implants, Congress passed the Medical Device Amendment of the Drug, Food and Cosmetics Act, setting up a separate section of the FDA to regulate and control medical devices such as sutures, heart valves, hip and knee joints, and intraocular lenses. Prior to this time the FDA was concerned mainly with drugs; because of the plethora of artificial devices, the FDA rightly wanted to assess their safety and effectiveness. Congress did not suspend the use of intraocular lenses, but asked that they be made "reasonably available" on an "investigational basis" to physicians meeting "appropriate qualifications."

It was not until February 9, 1978, that the FDA study of intraocular lenses began. It was probably the largest clinical FDA study ever devised, compiling data on almost a million implants from 1978 through 1985. The FDA hoped to amass enough data to make a definitive decision on the safety and effectiveness of intraocular lenses. Surgeon and patient alike had to meet several FDA requirements before an implant could be performed:

1. All ophthalmologists who wanted to implant intraocular lenses must have assisted at implant surgery and developed the necessary skills for this specialized operation. They must have registered separately with each company whose implants they wanted to insert.

2. Because many intraocular lenses were under investigation, patients had to sign a consent form that explained the risks of intraocular lenses. More and more implants have been approved for use as enough data accumulated to demonstrate their safety. Today, approved implants are available to any ophthalmologist regardless of training and patients no longer have to sign a special consent form.

3. After intraocular lens surgery, patients had to receive an identification card showing what type of implant was inserted, the name of the manufacturer, date of surgery, and name of the surgeon. Should patients move or need medical care when traveling, they will have a record of the implant. A copy of this card is also sent to the manufacturer, who can notify patients should any problems arise with the particular type of implant.

4. Any adverse reactions, however rare they may be, such as infection or severe inflammation, must be immediately reported to the manufacturer, whose records are periodically reviewed by the FDA.

On December 1, 1981, almost four years after this massive study began, the Choyce Mark VIII and IX anterior chamber implants by Coburn Optical Industries became the first intraocular lenses to be taken off investigational status by the FDA and approved for general use. These implants have since been replaced by many others of improved design.

Several implants are still under investigation, such as bifocal implants and advanced foldable implants. The field of implants is constantly changing. Standard implants, once thought to be "state-of-the-art," are being replaced by newer ones of improved design. Of the six implant companies listed in the first edition of this book, only one is still in existence, and of the two dozen implants listed, none is in active use today. Some of the more common companies and implants of today are:

ALCON SURGICAL (Fort Worth, Texas)
• Anterior Chamber Implant (MTAU)
• Posterior Chamber Implants (models MZ-20BD, MZ60BD, MZ30BD)

ALLERGAN MEDICAL OPTICS (Santa Ana, California)
• Posterior Chamber Implants (phacoFlex SI-26NB, PC-36NB, PC-43NB)

IOLAB CORPORATION (A Johnson & Johnson Company) (Claremont, California)
• Anterior Chamber Implant
• Posterior Chamber Implants (Formflex, Slimfit 3841S, 4897B, 8591B, 8191B)

IOPTEX RESEARCH (Irwindale, California)
• Anterior Chamber Implant (AP961)

• Posterior Chamber Implants (UPB350S, UPB260S, UPB350FNS, UPB320GS

KABI PHARMACIA OPHTHALMICS (Monrovia, California)
• Posterior Chamber Implant (810F, 815A, 722D, UB120)

OPTICAL RADIATION CORPORATION (Azusa, California)
• Posterior Chamber Implants (C41F, C430M)

STORZ OPHTHALMICS (Clearwater, Florida)
• Anterior Chamber Implant (121UV)
• Posterior Chamber Implants (Capsulorlens P359UV, P337UV, P390UV)

SURGIDEV CORPORATION (Goleta, California)
• Posterior Chamber Implants (SBUV, 5BUV, 6BUV)

3M VISION CARE (St. Paul, Minnesota)
• Posterior Chamber Implants (52X, 55X)

Implants that are still "investigational" are not necessarily less safe than those off investigational status. It is generally just a matter of time before the FDA reviews enough data for each lens, after which the implant is made freely available to all ophthalmologists and their patients. Your ophthalmologist will have up-to-date information on all intraocular lenses. Newer lenses, such as the bifocal or multifocal implant and new foldable implants, should be available in late 1993 or early 1994.

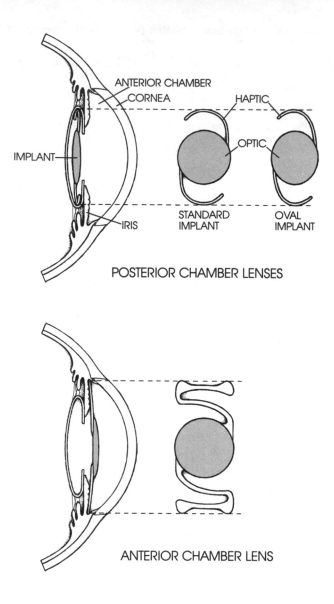

ANTERIOR CHAMBER
CORNEA
HAPTIC
OPTIC
IMPLANT
IRIS
STANDARD
IMPLANT
OVAL
IMPLANT

POSTERIOR CHAMBER LENSES

ANTERIOR CHAMBER LENS

Figure 9   Anterior and posterior chamber implants.

Given this background, we should discuss the implant itself, the source of a raging controversy years ago and now the source of vision restoration to countless millions of people throughout the world. What is an implant?

An implant is a small, clear plastic lens of a certain power or prescription inserted into the eye just after the cataract is removed. It replaces the human lens and helps the cornea focus light onto the retina to give a clear image. All implants have two main parts, a haptic and an optic. The optic is the center of the implant, usually 6 or 7 millimeters or about 1/4 inch in diameter, and is made of either PMMA, the same material as the Spitfire canopy, or of silicone. The optic is the optical part of the implant; it focuses the image onto the retina. The haptic acts as a spring and holds the implant in place. The magnification that results from an implant is only 1 percent, a negligible amount. It gives the closest approximation to normal vision possible today. Although there are about fifteen different implant companies manufacturing over one hundred different implants, all implants fall into three general categories based on their location in the eye. (See Fig. 9.)

ANTERIOR CHAMBER IMPLANTS

These implants are inserted into the fluid-filled space between the iris and cornea, the anterior chamber. The optic, or center, of the implant lies just in front of the pupil, and the haptics of the implant are lodged into the angle between the iris and cornea, fixating the implant so it cannot move. This is the second most common implant used today.

POSTERIOR CHAMBER IMPLANTS

These implants are placed behind the iris in the posterior chamber, the space between the iris and the vitreous. The haptics either lodge in a crevice behind the iris called the ciliary sulcus or fit into the lens capsule, occupying the exact position of the original cataract. This is the most commonly used intraocular lens.

IRIS-SUPPORTED IMPLANTS

These lenses were quite popular in the late 1970s and gave good results, but are now almost obsolete due to the

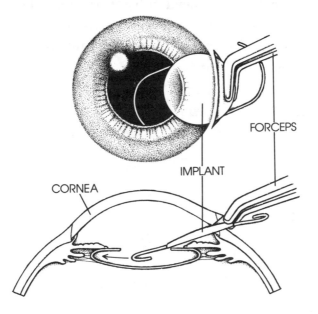

Figure 10   Insertion of a posterior chamber implant.

higher chance of inflammation. Iris-supported lenses are either sewn or clipped to the iris so that they do not move inside the eye. The original iris-supported lens, the Binkhorst lens, worked well, but improvements in the anterior and posterior chamber lenses have led to its demise.

Although an intracapsular cataract extraction with an anterior chamber implant gave excellent results in the 1970s, there is no doubt today that to most closely mimic the eye's natural lens, the procedure of choice is extracapsular cataract surgery or phacoemulsification with a posterior chamber implant.

The Posterior Chamber Implant

Two main types of posterior chamber implants are available: those more suitable to standard extracapsular cataract surgery and those modified and used for phacoemulsification. Whichever implant is used, the technique of intraocular lens insertion is almost the same, occurring during cataract surgery just after the cataract is removed. The implant is usually coated with a protective layer of a viscoelastic like Healon, lest it rub against the cornea, and is inserted into the eye and nudged into place. Stitches, if used, aid in sealing the wound closed, and the operation is essentially over (see Fig. 10).

In the last chapter we learned about a new method of extracapsular surgery, phacoemulsification with a small tunnel incision. Although this allowed eye surgeons to almost magically remove a 9-millimeter cataract through a 3-millimeter opening, the incision had to be enlarged to permit the insertion of a standard, round 6 or 7-millimeter implant, thus losing some of the advantages of the small tunnel incision. Eye surgeons had come close to perfecting small-incision cataract surgery by phacoemulsification, but were forced to implant lenses requiring larger incisions. Oval and foldable lenses are two implant innovations that complement small-incision cataract surgery. The oval PMMA implant, developed by Dr. Henry Clayman of Miami, Florida, and later adopted by many implant companies, measures 5 by 6 millimeters rather than the standard, round 6 or 7 millimeters of most implants. (See Fig. 9.) The oval 5- by 6-millimeter shape permits the surgeon to insert the implant through a 5-millimeter rather than a standard 7-millimeter incision. Even though the 5-millimeter incision is larger than the 3 millimeters needed for phacoemulsification, rapid healing and little or no astigmatism still result. The foldable implant, made of silicone, and developed by American Medical Optics (AMO), was even more remarkable. The flexibility of silicone allowed the 6-millimeter implant to be folded in half and inserted through a 4-millimeter incision. The surgeon first would use forceps (tweezers) to fold the implant and ease it through the incision. (See Fig. 11.) As the forceps were slowly opened, the implant was guided into place in the cocoon-like capsular bag, occupying the same position as did the cataract. The capsular bag, the space between the back (posterior) and front (anterior) parts of the lens capsule, helps center the intraocular lens in place and in effect isolates the implant from the rest of the eye, resulting in less inflammation and faster healing.

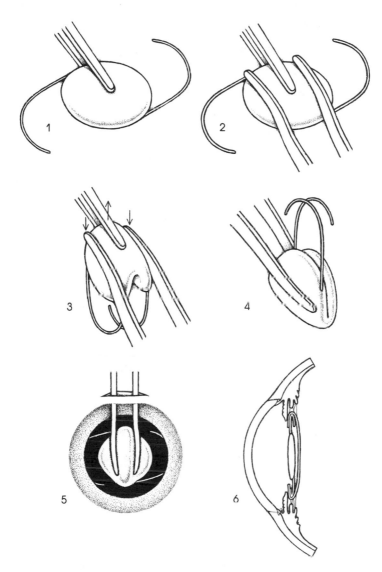

Figure 11   Insertion of a foldable implant.

Oval and foldable implants evolved out of a need for small-incision implants to maintain the advantages of small-incision surgery. Ophthalmologists disagree about the use of standard 6- or 7-millimeter implants in small-incision surgery; many maintain that a standard implant and a slightly larger incision give equally good results as do small incisions. Why use the relatively new oval implants, whose edge may give a slightly higher chance of glare, or go through the mechanical olympics of folding and unfolding a silicone implant? Certainly, if your eye surgeon prefers regular extracapsular surgery rather than small-incision phacoemulsification, or if your cataract is too advanced for phacoemulsification, a standard implant is best for you. If you are scheduled for small-incision surgery, you will have to leave the choice of implant in the hands of your surgeon, since his or her judgment will be your best guide. Whether you have a standard implant or an oval or foldable one, after reading this chapter you will certainly be better able to discuss your options. If nothing else, you can startle your ophthalmologist by asking if your cataract will be removed by phacoemulsification using a tunnel incision and a foldable silicone implant or by regular extracapsular surgery with a standard PMMA 7-millimeter implant!

As miraculous as is exchanging your cataractous human lens for a clear plastic one, there are times when an implant is either inadvisable or not possible. In the first edition of this book I provided guidelines for deciding on an implant. These guidelines, reproduced from Dr. Norman Jaffe's *Cataract Surgery and Its Complications* (St. Louis: C.V.

Mosby Co., 1976), reflected the conservative attitude of ophthalmologists toward the relatively new field of implants. Now we no longer restrict implants to patients over age sixty-five nor do we advise against an implant in a patient with only one eye. Severe diabetes and glaucoma are no longer contraindications for a well-performed posterior chamber implant. Several special situations do exist, however, that will affect whether or not you receive an implant. The most common situation is when you are extremely nearsighted, or myopic. The more nearsighted you are before cataract surgery, the weaker will be your eyeglass correction after surgery, since a nearsighted eye has too much refracting power and taking out the lens markedly reduces the refracting power. The A-scan ultrasound test will estimate what implant power your surgeon should choose, in preparation for a desired eyeglass prescription. This is about the only time in your life when you can have some input into the strength of your own prescription. Most eye surgeons will recommend making you slightly nearsighted, so that without glasses you can still read and yet see distance fairly well. Glasses will usually be necessary to fine-tune your vision for near and far, despite having an intraocular lens. Vision without glasses is a trade off—the better your vision is for distance, the more you will need glasses for reading, and vice versa.

If the ultrasound estimate shows that an implant power of close to zero will leave you needing glasses hardly at all, it may not make sense to have an implant. Patients whose refractive error is -15.00 diopters or more generally fall into this category. Although very safe, implants are not free of complications, as we will see in Chapter 10. The A-scan test will guide the ophthalmologist in selecting the most suitable intraocular lens power for your needs.

Patients who had cataract surgery in one eye years ago, without an implant, and are now ready for surgery in the other eye, are presented with a unique situation. To benefit from vision of an implant, patients should realize that after surgery, cataract glasses cannot be used. Patients would see double due to the imbalance between an implant in one eye and thick cataract glasses in the other. Some ophthalmologists would recommend an implant in the second eye, followed by fitting the first eye with a contact lens or, several months later, performing a secondary implant in that first eye. In a secondary implant operation, which is usually briefer than a cataract operation, an implant is inserted into an eye that has already had its cataract removed, but without an intraocular lens replacement. It is very successful and gives results equal to the more common primary implant operation, one in which the implant is inserted at the time of cataract surgery. Some of my most grateful patients have been those who have struggled for years with thick cataract glasses or contact lenses only to have natural sight restored by a secondary implant. Your ophthalmologist can determine if a secondary implant will help you.

In rare instances, the planned and expected insertion of an implant at the time of "routine" cataract surgery is impossible or dangerous. This situation occurs when the eye lacks enough space to safely accommodate the implant. When the cataract is removed, either by extracapsular surgery or phacoemulsification, the back membrane of the cataract, the posterior capsule, remains in the eye, acting like a cellophane barrier between the front of the eye and the vitreous in the back of the eye. In some instances, during surgery the vitreous moves forward and obliterates the space occupied by the cataract and reserved for the implant. Your eye surgeon can handle this situation, called vitreous pressure, in a number of ways. One way is to use Healon or other viscoelastics to increase the space needed for the implant. If there is still not enough room, the implant will have to be abandoned and the operation finished. The patient will either wear a contact lens or have a secondary implant later on. Vitreous pressure is much less common in a secondary implant.

In other instances, during surgery a tear develops in the thin posterior capsule, allowing the vitreous to creep forward like honey spreading from a cracked jar. With "vitreous loss," as this is called by ophthalmologists, an implant is still possible but only after the vitreous is removed by an instrument that acts like a suction cutter. In most cases of vitreous loss, either a posterior chamber or anterior chamber implant can still be inserted.

Even more rarely, bleeding can occur in the back of the eye, forcing your eye surgeon to finish the operation as quickly as possible so that the bleeding stops. An implant may have to be aborted for the safety of your eye, and inserted later as a secondary implant.

Although almost every patient scheduled to have cataract surgery with an implant will wind up with one, unforeseen or uncontrollable events can happen during surgery that make it more prudent not to insert an implant. Vitreous pressure and vitreous loss are unlikely, but should they occur during surgery, your ophthalmologist can usually safely insert an implant. Cataract and implant surgery is still one of the most successful operations performed on the human body.

9

Recovery: The Postoperative Period

The postoperative period starts as soon as you leave the operating room and lasts until your eye is completely healed. It can take as little as one or two weeks or as long as three or four months. It is an exciting period, during which your vision gradually improves. When your eye doctor removes the patch from your eye during your first postoperative visit, your vision may surprise you: It may be amazingly clear or amazingly poor, even worse than before surgery. If your cataract blocked most of your vision before surgery, your vision may, in comparison, seem "perfect" the day after surgery and will probably improve even further over the next month. However, due to normal inflammation and clouding of the cornea and even temporary transient bleeding, vision can be temporarily worse for the first few days or even weeks after surgery. Vision improvement almost invariably follows, and all your doctor needs is a brief look at your eye to reassure you all is in order. No matter how many times I've removed the patch on that first postoperative day, I never get over the thrill of seeing a patient's eye for the first time after surgery.

Reactions to Surgery

During the postoperative period you will probably experience some of the following reactions to your surgery.

PAIN

Cataract surgery can lead to as great a variety of symptoms as there are people. Some pain is normal, but what may be annoying pain for one person may be a trifling discomfort for another. Postoperative pain is usually mild and is relieved by nonprescription pain medication. It is a good idea to avoid aspirin, which can sometimes promote bleeding. Most local anesthetics will wear off a few hours after surgery, unless your ophthalmologist used a longer-acting anesthetic, which can last eight to twelve hours. By the evening of surgery, your pain will usually be only a mild aching and should not prevent a normal night's sleep. A foreign body sensation, as if you had an eyelash in your eye, is also common and is a normal reaction to the surgery. This also should clear in a day or so. Severe pain is quite unusual and should be reported to your doctor promptly.

FLOATERS AND FLASHES

For several days, weeks, or even months after cataract surgery, you may see black spots or other shapes in your line of sight or off to one side. You may even think you see a fly or bug, only to see it disappear on turning your head. A flash of light may appear off to the side like a streak of lightning or the discharge of a flashbulb. These are very common symptoms and stem from changes in the vitreous. After the cataract is removed, the vitreous will tend to shrink away from the back of the eye and move toward the front, taking up some of the space occupied by the cataract. This movement often releases debris or clumps of vitreous gel we see as black spots or lines. Floaters were even known in ancient times. The Romans called them muscae volitantes, or "flying flies," for obvious reasons. If the vitreous pulls on the retina, to which it is loosely attached, it may stimulate the retina just as light does on entering the eye, fooling you into thinking you see a flash of light.

On very rare occasions the movement of the vitreous away from the retina may pull off a piece and cause a retinal tear and a detached retina. Fluid from inside the eye will flow through the tear, travel behind the retina, and peel it off like old wallpaper. About 1 to 2 percent of all patients undergoing cataract surgery develop a torn retina no matter how successful the surgery or how skilled the surgeon. This may happen weeks, months, or even years afterward. Periodic checkups can detect the torn retina before the detachment starts, allowing repair by a simple laser treatment rather than an actual operation.

Symptoms of a torn retina are similar to those of vitreous floaters, such as seeing spots and flashes of light. These symptoms will, in the vast majority of cases, indicate merely vitreous floaters and not a detached retina. Your eye doctor will be able to differentiate the two during an office visit.

TEARING AND DISCHARGE

These are common nonspecific symptoms through which the eye is voicing some protest over being disturbed. The tearing should be quite mild and should require nothing more than a gentle dab with a clean tissue. The discharge, mainly mucus production, will be present mostly in the morning on awakening and should be gently wiped away with a clean wet tissue or gauze. If tearing and discharge is anything more than mild, contact your ophthalmologist.

DROOPY LID

Many patients will have some swelling and drooping of the upper lid. This *ptosis* (pronounced "toesis"), as eye doctors call the droopy lid, is a normal reaction to the inflammation from the surgery and generally disappears in a few weeks. Infrequently the droopy lid lasts for several months and rarely, permanently.

LIGHT SENSITIVITY

Naturally more light will be entering your eye after the cataract is removed, and you may find it slightly uncomfortable until you adapt to this change. The iris, the colored part of your eye, constricts to light, and the normal inflammation in the iris after surgery makes this constriction feel uncomfortable. As the eye becomes less inflamed it will become much less light sensitive. Although most implants contain an ultraviolet filter, a good pair of sunglasses will be necessary to eliminate any remaining discomfort from bright light.

Glare, another form of light sensitivity due to light scattering as it enters the eye, may be annoying, especially when driving at night. Often due to light reflecting off the implant or the posterior capsule, glare decreases over several weeks or months. Occasionally some glare may be permanent.

RESTRICTION OF ACTIVITY

Restriction of activity after a well-performed cataract extraction will vary greatly, depending on the judgment of your doctor. Sixty years ago, before the development of sutures for cataract surgery, there was nothing with which to close the incision into the eye, and the patient had to lie almost immobile for weeks while the incision healed enough to permit any activity—even getting up to eat and go to the bathroom. If activity began too soon, the wound might open and fluid inside the eye would leak out, inviting infection and glaucoma. Modern-day surgical techniques result in a tightly closed wound, and most surgeons permit almost normal activity the day after surgery. This is true whether you had a small incision with phacoemulsification with or without sutures, or the somewhat larger incision with an extracapsular cataract opera-

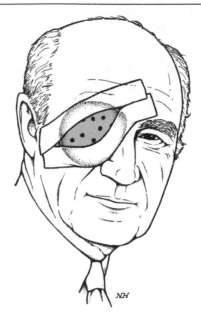

Figure 12   Correct way to wear the shield and tape.

tion. I permit my own patients to bend, lift, read, shower, and do all of their usual daily activities right after surgery. At bedtime a plastic or metal shield is taped over the eye to protect it, lest you rub it or lie on it during sleep. (See Fig. 12.) This is usually necessary for several weeks, but with phacoemulsification the incision is so small that a shield may be needed only for a few days, if at all. Be sure to follow your own doctor's advice.

REDNESS

Your eye will be red and look inflamed for several weeks after surgery. This can look quite frightening, but the redness quickly disappears as the eye heals.

DOUBLE VISION

Double vision (diplopia) is usually normal and transitory after cataract surgery. An eye with a dense cataract and limited vision for several years can drift, and once vision is restored the eye has to learn to work with the other eye again. Until that occurs, the eyes will be misaligned, resulting in double vision. Unequal refractive errors of your eyes, such as one eye being nearsighted and one eye farsighted, and inflammation of one of the eye's six muscles may also cause double vision until your eye heals. Rarely, double vision can be permanent, requiring special prism glasses or even eye muscle surgery to control it.

Medication and Office Visits

After cataract surgery your ophthalmologist will prescribe certain eyedrops and medications. The following are the most common ones.

CORTISONE (STEROID)

After any type of cataract operation, there will be a certain amount of inflammation inside the eye. With the aid of magnification from the slit lamp, your ophthalmologist can see the inflammation as tiny white blood cells floating in the aqueous fluid of your eye. The slit beam of light passing through the fluid will show a smoky appearance, like real smoke in a darkened theater when it drifts into the beam of the movie projector. The more white blood cells in the aqueous fluid, the more the inflammation and the smokier the light will appear. Cortisone and other steroid eyedrops are used to clear up this inflammation, which generally lasts from four to six weeks with extracapsular cataract surgery and two to three weeks with phacoemulsification. The word cortisone often makes people uneasy, because significant side effects can occur when the drug is taken by mouth. In eyedrop form, however, cortisone has virtually no general side effects and is extremely effective not only in aiding healing but in quickly alleviating any symptoms of discomfort.

ANTIBIOTICS

Antibiotic drops are often given for several weeks in the belief that they will lessen the minuscule chance of infection. Antibiotic drops are actually more effective in preventing infection when given just before surgery rather than after, but it is common to use them in the postoperative period on the theory that "it can't hurt." Many eye surgeons will inject an antibiotic on the inside of the lower lid at the very end of surgery, since this does help lessen the chance of infection. The injection may cause some soreness and swelling in the area, making your eye look more inflamed and red than it really is. This disappears in a few days. A common practice is to prescribe a single eyedrop that combines cortisone and antibiotics, so that the patient will not have to use two separate drops.

DILATING DROPS

Drops that open the pupils, such as Mydriacyl and Cyclogyl, are used before surgery to allow easier access to

the cataract, and sometimes after surgery to fight inflammation, alleviate discomfort, and prevent the iris from
adhering to the implant. Most ophthalmologists will use
dilating drops after surgery only when more than the usual
inflammation is present.

DROPS TO LOWER INTRAOCULAR PRESSURE

The pressure inside the eye may rise for the first few
days or weeks after cataract surgery, and drops called beta-
blockers, such as Timoptic, or pills such as Diamox may
be needed to lower the pressure. Glaucoma, a disease in
which elevated eye pressure damages the delicate optic
nerve, rarely develops after cataract surgery. In fact, patients with glaucoma will often be surprised to learn that
their elevated eye pressure is actually easier to control
after cataract surgery.

The day after surgery, your ophthalmologist will check
the progress of healing and improvement in vision. Most
of the tests performed then will be identical to those performed prior to surgery, but now you will have the excite-
ment of reading the eye chart with your operated eye. If
you are a bit disappointed, do not worry; your vision may
still be blurred from inflammation inside the eye, a cloudy
cornea, and a lot of astigmatism arising from irregular
healing of the cornea. All of this should subside over the
next few weeks, and your vision will improve daily. This
first postoperative visit is intended more to detect any
complications than to fully examine your eye.

After you read the eye chart as far down as you can, a
brief refraction will be performed to get your best corrected

vision. An implant will allow you to see moderately well within a few days of cataract surgery, and the refraction will show you how much further improvement you will get with glasses.

After the refraction the doctor will examine your eye under the slit lamp, check your intraocular pressure, and perhaps examine your retina. This will be the doctor's first clear view into your eye since you developed the cataract, and he or she will be able to tell you if your retina is healthy or not. About 10 percent of patients with cataracts also have retina trouble in the form of macular degeneration, an aging change of the center of the retina (the macula). Patients with healthy retinas will have almost no impediment to normal vision. In those patients with macular degeneration, vision will undoubtedly be better than before surgery but not as good as if the retina were normal. Macular degeneration affects reading vision more than distance vision.

The number of postoperative visits will depend on the progress of healing of your eye, whether you had extracapsular surgery or phacoemulsification, and the philosophy of your doctor. With extracapsular cataract extraction, most doctors feel comfortable with three or four checkups over the next six weeks; others may want to see you almost every week to ensure early detection of any complications. By your sixth postoperative week your eye should generally be free of redness and should feel comfortable. Some additional healing and change may occur up to six months later, but in general, six to eight postoperative weeks is the time for your final refraction and glasses.

With phacoemulsification, only two or three visits are necessary, since healing is usually complete by three weeks.

Even after having an implant, chances are you will still need glasses to correct any remaining near- or farsightedness or astigmatism and to fine-tune either your distance or near vision to its maximum.

If a lot of astigmatism is present, due to one or two tight sutures or unequal healing of the incision, your doctor will probably want to remove the sutures and allow the cornea to return to a more normal, rounded shape. This takes a few seconds at the slit lamp and is painless with an anesthetic eyedrop. Should this be necessary, you will have to wait another one to two weeks before getting glasses to allow your cornea to change to a more normal shape. Be patient, as you are the one to ultimately benefit. The less astigmatism you have after cataract surgery, the clearer and more comfortable will be your vision.

Contact Lens Fitting

Although fewer than 1 percent of patients need a contact lens after cataract surgery, problems during surgery, such as severe bleeding or severe vitreous pressure, may make it impossible or imprudent to insert an implant. A contact lens would then be needed to restore sight fully. Before the era of intraocular lenses, a contact lens was the most popular way to restore sight after cataract surgery. Soft lenses are quite comfortable and can be worn continuously for a week or longer. Although an implant is preferable, contact lenses are very successful in most patients, even first-time wearers in their seventies and eighties. If not, a secondary implant can be performed several months after the original surgery. Your eye doctor will guide you through the process of contact lens fitting and will be able to judge whether a second operation to insert an implant would be advisable. Many contact lens wearers who undergo cataract surgery with an implant but are left more nearsighted or farsighted than they'd like can be refit with a new contact lens and resume wear after the eye has healed.

Once you are wearing your new glasses, or possibly a contact lens, and your doctor has told you he doesn't have to see you for four, five, or even six months, your postoperative period is over. Barring any eye problems such as retina or cornea trouble or glaucoma, you should now be able to read and drive a lot easier, watch television, and do all the other things you enjoy. If retina trouble such as macular degeneration is present, the improvement in your vision will be limited, but some should occur. Significant retina trouble may require you to use low-vision aids such as magnifying glasses, high-intensity lighting, and telescopic devices to supplement the improvement from your cataract operation.

10

Complications

The old adage "Doctors are human" pertains to all surgery, including cataract surgery. Although some complications can be ascribed to doctor error, most are not and stem from unusual circumstances during surgery beyond the control of your doctor. It is a question of statistics and bad luck—if doctors do surgery, eventually they will encounter complications. Most complications are unlikely to occur and are usually not serious, but some rare complications can result in loss of vision and even loss of the eye. All these complications are extremely unlikely but should be mentioned to complete your understanding of cataracts and cataract surgery. Again, all of the following complications are unlikely to happen.

Vitreous Loss

This was mentioned on p. 123 and occurs when, during cataract removal, some vitreous flows from the back of the eye through the pupil, into the front of the eye. Modern surgical technique and instrumentation enable your doctor to remove the vitreous safely with a cutting and suction instrument so that now, unlike years ago, glaucoma and retinal detachment are much less likely to occur with vitreous loss. If vitreous loss does occur, your doctor may decide to use an anterior chamber implant in front of the iris, rather than a posterior chamber implant behind the iris. Since the posterior capsule is usually torn with vitreous loss, it may be too weak to support a posterior chamber implant, making an anterior chamber implant a better choice. Most operating rooms stock a complete inventory of posterior and anterior chamber implants in a variety of powers. The nurse has only to hand the surgeon the desired implant in the event a substitute is needed during the operation itself. Vision should recover completely or almost so.

Cystoid Macular Edema (CME)

This refers to the leakage of fluid from tiny capillaries in the macula, the center of the retina. The exact cause of CME is not known, but it is thought that excessive inflammation can lead to the accumulation of fluid in the center of the macula. CME can occur after the most perfect cataract operation and is treated by anti-inflammatory eyedrops or even a cortisone injection near the eye. Recovery is usually complete, although some permanent reduction in vision may remain.

Cloudy Cornea

As I mentioned on p. 00, the delicate cells lining the back of the cornea keep it clear by preventing aqueous fluid in the front of the eye from entering the cornea and causing it to be swollen and cloudy. These cells tend to weaken with age, and are less able to keep the cornea clear after the normal trauma of cataract surgery. If the cornea does get cloudy after surgery, medication usually is successful in restoring clarity. Corneal clouding may sometimes require a corneal transplant to restore clarity.

Decentered Implant

Weakness or excessive scarring of the posterior capsule can, on rare occasions, cause decentering of the implant. Although it is not necessary for the implant to be perfectly centered to achieve good vision, since the size of the central part, the optic, is generous enough to allow for slight shifts, too much movement of the implant will cause blurred and distorted vision. This problem occurs in less than 1 percent of cataract operations but may require a second operation to reposition the implant or to exchange it for another.

Bleeding

During the typical cataract operation, there is almost no bleeding, and even patients on blood thinners, such as Coumadin, can safely have surgery. Occasionally there is slight bleeding in the front of the eye that mixes with the aqueous fluid; this may cause blurred vision for several days after surgery until the blood washes out of the eye with the normal flow of aqueous. During surgery, bleeding of a much more serious nature can occur in the back of the eye, in the choroid, the area rich in blood vessels behind the retina. This bleeding can cause severe vitreous loss, a detached retina, and total loss of vision. Fortunately, your eye doctor can usually stop the bleeding during surgery to minimize any permanent damage. This type of bleeding is extremely rare.

Anesthesia

In order to be effective, the local anesthetic must be injected somewhat close to and behind (retrobulbar) the eye. Since your eye doctor cannot see the tip of the needle once it is past the skin of the eyelid, he or she must control the path of the needle by feel. Fortunately, this type of local anesthesia is quite accurate and safe. Very rarely will the needle damage the eye or the optic nerve behind it.

Many ophthalmologists have adopted a new technique called peribulbar anesthesia; it is less likely to cause damage because the injection is given a bit farther away from the eye. Local anesthesia is extremely safe.

Infection

This is one of the most dreaded complications of cataract surgery, occurring in 1 out of about 50,000 operations. No matter how sterile the operating room, how thoroughly the nurse washes the area around your eye, and how many precautions are taken to prevent infection, a few germs can still find their way into your eye during surgery. Almost invariably, your own immune system and the antibiotic solutions given during surgery will kill these germs. Very rarely some germs will survive, and over several days or weeks after surgery an infection can occur in your eye, causing severe inflammation and loss of vision. Although a second operation is usually successful in halting the infection, permanent damage can occur. If the infection cannot be controlled with antibiotics, the eye may even have to be removed. Like all the other complications already discussed, this is extremely rare and is a nightmare for patient and doctor alike.

All surgery has some risk, and with cataract surgery the risk is very small. Despite these unlikely and rare complications, cataract surgery remains one of the most successful operations performed on the human body.

11

Lasers and Cataract Surgery

I am frequently asked by patients if their cataract will be removed by laser or if I perform "laser cataract surgery." When I quickly answer "no," I often see looks of surprise and shades of doubt, since many patients assume phaco-emulsification is laser surgery. Lasers are definitely *not* used to remove a cataract at least not at the time of this writing. Although researchers are studying the use of lasers in cataract surgery, and several prototypes have been produced, there is little evidence to suggest any significant development in this area for several years.

The word laser is actually an acronym for Light Amplification by Stimulated Emission of Radiation. A laser beam is what physicists call coherent light—that is, it is made up of light waves closely packed together and all traveling in the same direction. This uniformity of light rays concentrates a tremendous amount of energy into a laser beam and gives the laser its power to cut tissue.

Although lasers are not used to remove cataracts, they are used to fine-tune vision after cataract surgery. About 20 to 30 percent of patients develop clouding of the posterior capsule, the thin back membrane of the original cataract that is purposely left in the eye at the end of cataract surgery. This clouding can reduce vision months or even years after cataract surgery and can have the same effect as if the cataract grew back. A simple YAG laser treatment, using energy from a crystal of yttrium aluminum garnet, will create a small opening in the center of the capsule,

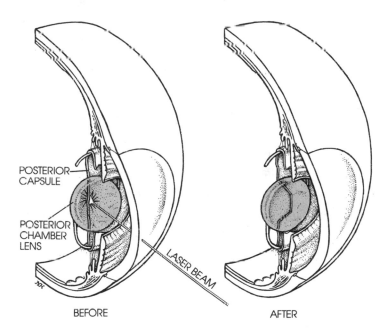

BEFORE   AFTER

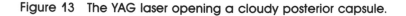

Figure 13   The YAG laser opening a cloudy posterior capsule.

restoring vision almost immediately. The 500,000-watt burst of laser energy, focused to a minute point on the center of the posterior capsule, lasts only a trillionth of a second but is all that is needed to open the capsule. (See Fig.13.) Before the advent of the YAG laser, this capsule had to be opened surgically. Although the operation was quite simple, it still carried some risk. YAG laser surgery can be performed painlessly and quickly in your doctor's office or in a hospital.

Although a YAG laser capsulotomy, as the procedure is called, is extremely safe, there is one drawback. Cataract surgery does increase the chances of a detached retina by one or two percentage points, and an intact, unlasered posterior capsule tends to reduce this slight risk. Even after the most perfect cataract operation, there is a slight risk of a detached retina occurring during the patient's lifetime. An intact posterior capsule tends to keep this risk at the 1 or 2 percent level, while an opened capsule, such as after a YAG laser treatment, tends to increase the risk to about 2 or 3 percent. Patients with reduced vision from a cloudy posterior capsule have no choice but to have a YAG laser treatment to restore sight, and the chances of retina trouble are still quite small. If a detached retina does occur, surgery is quite successful in repairing the detachment. Several researchers from Houston Biotechnology Incorporated have developed a chemical to be used at the end of cataract surgery that promises to inhibit and greatly reduce the clouding of the posterior capsule. Clinical trials are expected in late 1993.

We have now surveyed the current state of our knowledge and skills in dealing with cataracts and the optical correction of the eye without its own natural lens. Ten or twenty years from now our current techniques may all seem primitive, but by keeping abreast of advances in the field of cataracts and implants, your ophthalmologist will be in an excellent position to give you the best care possible. Let's see what the future may hold.

12

What the Future Holds

The burden of cataract blindness throughout the world is enormous, and although cataract surgery has been practiced for many years, cataracts remain the major cause of blindness worldwide, affecting about 50 million people. In undeveloped countries such as India, there are just not enough eye surgeons to treat the cataract population, and although cataract camps where hundreds of cataract operations are done every day alleviate the immediate local problem, many cataract patients around the world go blind from a treatable disease. To further illustrate the enormity of the cataract problem worldwide, in England and Wales alone in 1988 there were a total of 66,000 people on ophthalmic waiting lists for surgery, mostly for cataract surgery. In the United States, where our health-care system is not socialized, there is little or no waiting list for cataract surgery. Although a good deal of cataract research will involve trying to refine and improve surgical results, most research energy will be expended searching for ways to develop anticataract drugs and to prevent cataracts from forming.

Prevention and Nonsurgical Treatment of Cataracts

According to a 1992 United States government panel report on the management of functional impairment due to cataract, there is no medical treatment to prevent or halt the progression of a cataract; nor is there any way to reverse a cataract once it has formed. The only known treatment is surgical. Although this will be true for some time, a great deal of research is underway to discover an alternative—a medical treatment for cataracts, such as a pill or an eyedrop to clear up the clouded lens. Research formally began in 1976, when twenty-three research laboratories throughout the United States agreed to pool their knowledge and resources into the Cooperative Cataract Research Group (CCRG). In 1980 this research was consolidated into seven centers with funding from the National Institutes of Health.

Before studying possible cures for cataracts, scientists have to learn how cataracts form and what makes them grow. Once this is known, anticataract drugs can be tested and the results evaluated. Research led by Dr. Clifford Harding, professor and director of research in ophthalmology at Kresge Institute in Detroit, and Dr. Leo T. Chylack,

Jr., of Harvard University and head of Boston's Cataract Research Center, has resulted in the examination and classification of thousands of human cataracts. This almost universally adopted classification will enable scientists from different countries to compare their results and share research so that more can be learned about cataract formation.

Dr. Abraham Spector of New York's Columbia University is doing research on an eyedrop that has the potential to neutralize the excess hydrogen peroxide found in cataracts and thought to cause their formation. Although many years remain before this anticataract eyedrop will be available to humans, results in laboratory experiments seem promising.

The most promising and immediate anticataract research concerns people with diabetes, in whom experimental drugs have already been developed to block the formation of cataracts from high blood sugar. These drugs easily block cataract formation in laboratory animals, but because of side effects clinical trials in humans were stopped. Since diabetes is fairly common, there is a multimillion-dollar impetus to develop a drug to prevent cataract formation in patients with diabetes. This will probably be a reality in ten to fifteen years.

Other drugs such as simple aspirin and ibuprofen have also been shown to protect the eye from developing a cataract, although how much protection these drugs afford is controversial. Studies in the United States and England showed that patients with rheumatoid arthritis who take aspirin and ibuprofen tend to have lower rates of cataract and develop cataracts at a later age. It is likely that large-scale clinical trials will be conducted in the United States to try to prove conclusively whether either drug should be taken to prevent or reduce the risk of cataract formation. It would be ironic if a simple drug such as aspirin, which has been shown to reduce the risk of heart attack and stroke, and is recommended for many cardiac patients, also reduces the risk of cataract formation.

Other substances, such as the antioxidants Vitamins C, E, and A, zinc, and selenium, are also being investigated for their protective effect against cataract formation. In a field like the study of vitamins and minerals and their role in disease prevention, there is always some danger in endorsing faddish solutions to age-old problems. But more and more hard evidence is accumulating that does show a place for nutritional strategy in preventing cataracts. Dr. Kailash Bhuyan, a cataract researcher at New York's Mount Sinai Hospital, in collaboration with its Chairman of Ophthalmology, Dr. Stephen M. Podos, has shown Vitamin E to inhibit the formation of cataracts in rabbits by about 50 percent. Vitamin E is probably our most potent antioxidant and protects the lens (and the heart and other organs) by deactivating harmful free radicals like hydrogen peroxide. Vitamins C and A and the minerals zinc and selenium are also beneficial, although somewhat less potent than Vitamin E.

Other studies also link nutrition to cataracts. The U.S. Department of Agriculture's Human Nutrition Research Center on Aging at Tufts University reported in 1991 that eating at least three and one-half servings of fruits and vegetables daily will make you five times less likely to develop cataracts than those who eat smaller amounts. Similar results have emerged in several studies conducted in the last few years; one report by researchers at the State University of New York (SUNY) at Stony Brook found patients who took vitamin supplements or regularly ate fruits and vegetables to be 30 percent less likely to develop cataracts.

Although the data is not yet conclusive, the evidence so far makes a strong case for nutritional supplements in helping to prevent cataracts. Some pharmaceutical companies have already begun to produce and market supplements in tablet form containing what are thought to be appropriate doses for antioxidant vitamins and minerals. Because the field of nutrition and cataracts is so new, no one really knows what an appropriate dose really is; but taking at least the Recommended Dietary Allowance (RDA) for each vitamin or mineral—whether through food, supplements, or both—should be a first step. The RDA for Vitamin E is 30 milligrams, for Vitamin C, 60 mg; and for Vitamin A, 5,000 IU (international units). E is most commonly found in grain-derived foods like oatmeal, wheat germ, peanut butter, brown rice, and nuts; Vitamin C is plentiful in fruits and vegetables—from sweet red peppers and broccoli to strawberries and papaya to, of course, orange juice. Vitamin A is plentiful in carrots, sweet potatoes, cantaloupe, and liver. Your ophthalmologist should offer you guidance in supplementing your diet with vitamins, minerals, and aspirin to reduce the risk of cataracts.

Wearing protective sunglasses to block ultraviolet light is another way to help minimize your chances of developing a cataract. Many ophthalmologists are now recommending that patients of all ages wear sunglasses to protect their eyes from ultraviolet rays, which are thought to create oxidative damage to the lens. Several studies, such as one 1988 study of 838 watermen working on Chesapeake Bay in significant ultraviolet exposure, did show a probable link between UV light and cataract formation. The role of ultraviolet light in cataract formation is still a subject of controversy, and is more widely accepted in the United States than in Great Britain, where the sunlight hypothesis has not received much support. Future studies are needed to determine whether wearing sunglasses will appreciably reduce your chances of getting a cataract.

Refractive Corneal Surgery

Refractive eye surgery generally refers to surgery to alter the shape of the cornea in an attempt to reduce myopia (nearsightedness) or astigmatism or both. In radial keratotomy (RK), the most common type of refractive surgery, microscopic slits are made in a symmetrical pattern on the surface of the cornea, like cuts in a pie, to flatten its overall curvature, resulting in less myopia. In a patient with astigmatism, astigmatic keratotomy (AK) is performed, in which these slits are placed asymmetrically to correspond to the asymmetrical curvature of the cornea. These days phacoemulsification has become so sophisticated and patient expectation so high that many eye surgeons, no longer content to merely do a perfect cataract operation, combine astigmatism surgery with cataract surgery to correct the entire optical problem of a cataract patient. By combining two or more tiny slits on the surface of the cornea with phacoemulsification, your ophthalmologist can increase your chances of the best vision possible and make you less dependent on glasses. Cataract removal and implant insertion will give you most of your vision improvement, while astigmatic keratotomy will fine-tune your vision. Astigmatism correction at the time of cataract surgery is still evolving, and will become more common in the mid- and late 1990s.

Excimer Laser

The excimer laser, a revolutionary advance in refractive eye surgery and slated for approval in the United States in 1995, will be another tool for ophthalmologists to use to improve their patients' vision. As we mentioned in Chapter 6, the ultrasound A-scan test is used to determine the implant power for each patient, so that most of the vision improvement will come from the implant and not from the supplementary use of glasses. Because the A-scan is not 100 percent accurate, some patients are left somewhat nearsighted or farsighted and must rely on glasses to see properly. For most patients this is more of an inconvenience than a problem, since normal vision with glasses is far better than the clouded vision of a cataract. Radial keratotomy as a second operation after cataract surgery would be an option in eliminating any residual myopia, but most patients would probably put up with the glasses rather than have a second operation.

The excimer laser would eliminate the need for radial keratotomy and would rely on light to correct excessive residual myopia and small amounts of astigmatism. Rather than making slits in the cornea as in radial keratotomy, your eye doctor will be able to use the concentrated light from the excimer laser to microscopically reshape your cornea, eliminating or greatly reducing myopia and mild astigmatism. Clinical studies, presently underway in the United States and abroad, are extremely promising. The excimer laser may very well have a tremendous impact on eye care, not only for cataract patients but also for the 90 million Americans who now wear glasses or contact lenses. Although some myopia after cataract surgery is often desired, since it will let you read without glasses, too much myopia may make you a candidate for the excimer laser. Check with your ophthalmologist if you would benefit from this remarkable development.

New Implants

Cataract surgery and the trend toward a smaller incision, such as in phacoemulsification, created a need for implants that could be inserted through the same small incision. The oval implant and the foldable silicone implant are two current examples, but others are on the way.

Compressable implants made of newer acrylics and other plastics will be able to fit through incisions as small as 2 or 3 millimeters and even 1 millimeter. Building a model ship in a bottle is a snap compared to what is on the horizon for cataract surgery. The result will be faster healing, possibly within one week, no astigmatism, and better vision. These implants should be available in 1993 or 1994.

More amazing than small-incision implants is the possibility of an implant that will have some of the focusing ability of the normally clear human lens. This may make it possible for a patient to do away with not only distance glasses after implant surgery but with reading glasses as well. Several companies are developing an implant that can be injected to expand and fill the space previously occupied by the cataract. The implant would then have some ability to change shape and therefore allow the patient to focus from distance to near without resorting to glasses. This implant is still in the research stage but may be a reality in a few years.

Well out of the research stage and almost a reality for all cataract patients are bifocal and multifocal implants, intraocular lenses that will make glasses unnecessary by providing not only good distance vision but good near and even midrange vision. Almost all of the more than twenty implant manufacturers in the United States are actively involved in developing their own implant, but most use either a bull's-eye design, where the center of the bull's-eye is focused for near and the outside for distance (or vice versa), or a diffractive design, where both distance and near are in focus and the brain selects whichever it needs. Results in several thousand patients have been excellent, especially in those with a bifocal implant in both eyes. Patient selection and realistic expectations are extremely important for success.

One of the main disadvantages to this technology is that some patients experience a loss of sharp contrast and image quality. Although this is usually not significant, any loss of image quality or contrast may not be advisable in patients with macular degeneration, severe glaucoma, or diabetes. Patients who prefer glasses out of habit or for cosmetic reasons and those who require extremely sharp vision at arm's length may also be unsuitable candidates for multifocal implants. But for those patients who hate glasses and do a lot of close work, the slight reduction in contrast may be a good trade-off for throwing away your glasses, possibly forever. As these implants get FDA pre-market approval and are made available to all ophthalmologists and their patients, implant companies will accumulate more data and results. The companies will provide this information to your ophthalmologist so that you and your doctor can decide if you are a good candidate.

The future for patients with cataracts has never been brighter. Not only are scientists doing pure academic research to discover the cause of cataracts and find a way to prevent their formation, but ophthalmologists, working on the other side of the problem, are perfecting ways of making the surgery more successful for their patients.

Even without these advances cataract surgery is one of the most successful of all operations. Except for the 10 percent of cataract patients who have retina trouble as well as cataracts, the chance of recovery of normal, clear vision after cataract surgery is over 95 percent. As advances continue, this high success rate will be even higher. The vast majority of patients will benefit from improved eyesight, better quality of life, and prevention of blindness. It is my hope that this book will help you attain these goals.

Index